# Diet Digest

## Grain Free Cooking and Anti Inflammation

Terri King and Beatrice Simmons

# Table of Contents

# Introduction

This Diet Digest book is just for people who suffer from inflammation issues. Inflammation is an area in the body that becomes swollen, reddened, and painful even due to an infection or injury. Inflammation can occur acutely due to sudden injury or infection. Chronic inflammation occurs as a result of certain health conditions like arthritis or from eating certain types of food like gluten. The inflammation occurs as a reaction, an attempt to protect the tissues from further infection or injury. While inflammation is a natural response of the immune system to help heal it can also cause other issues such as the pain and swelling. It is chronic inflammation that becomes the problem, when the body attempts to heal an area that just won't heal or the body won't stop the inflammation and it becomes chronic where the immune system response will not let up on it.

One of the best treatments for any health issue is to first try dieting. Food is nature's very own medicine cabinet. If we eat the right foods our body has nutrients to use to help fight infections and correct health issues. It is the first line of defense and should always be the first step to healing and prevention. The same holds true if we eat junk food we are putting zero nutrients into our body and only supplying it with sugars and fat. This will only serve to perpetuate any underlying illnesses. But if we go in the opposite direction and eat healthy foods we give our bodies a boost for healing. The Diet Digest book contains recipes that help to fight inflammation. Eating the foods in these recipes will help the body to heal and treat conditions that cause inflammation.

The body is remarkable in how it knows how to pull the right nutrients from the foods we eat and send them to the areas that needs it. What happens is when we eat healthy whole foods our body absorbs the nutrients, the vitamins, antioxidants, minerals, amino acids, and other healthy substances from the foods. The immune system is strengthened by these nutrients. When the immune system is strong and healthy it can aid the body in fighting off harmful illnesses. It can also prevent harmful health conditions from taking hold. Both the anti inflammatory diet and the grain free diets help the body to fight chronic inflammation.

If you suffer from chronic inflammation then you are making the right step to combating it with the recipes in this book. You can do things to further help you to feel better. Part of the reason why you suffer from chronic inflammation may have to do with the foods you currently eat. Are you addicted to junk foods? Do you consume a lot of sugars and fats? Do you eat "processed convenient" foods? These foods have very little real nutrition and if you already have chronic inflammation they will just aggravate the condition. By changing your diet you will help your body to truly heal and treat the inflammation issues. First, if you do have an addiction to junk foods you need to wean from this in order to set up for a successful dieting change.

Make the diet a healthy lifestyle change. You need to make it a permanent part of your every day routine. It is true that if you diet long enough you will find your inflammation issues my either go away completely or at least be better managed. But you do not want to get to this point only to fall back into your old eating habits and have the inflammation issues reoccur. It is a guarantee that if you do not make this a permanent change the old health issues will resurface and you will be right back where you began. Look at the diet as a positive step in the right direction to making a lifestyle change for the better.

First give yourself a good three weeks to break bad eating habits. It takes the body three weeks to overcome any habit and make the changes to the better habits. This is true of any habit, be it a smoking habit, a drinking alcohol habit, drugs, and eating junk food. In three weeks your body will wean from the junk food and you will be able to focus on eating healthy all the time without the terrible withdrawal symptoms you may have from weaning from junk food if you just suddenly stop. Withdrawal from junk food causes headaches, moodiness, and intense junk food cravings. You can avoid this by doing a slow three week wean. While you are in the three weeks eat the recipes from the Diet Digest as you wean from the junk food. This way you are helping your body to be used to eating the healthy foods.

The first week only eat junk food twice. The second week you will only eat junk food once a day. The third week you will go to eating junk food just once every other day. By the end of the third week you should be weaned from the junk food. If you still find you crave the junk food you can give yourself a "reward" of a junk food treat just once a week. Eventually you will no longer crave the junk. Eventually the healthy nutritious food you eat will keep you quite satisfied.

Once you make the lifestyle change stick with it. It is so much better for your health to be eating healthy nutritious foods. Your body will react by helping you to feel better. The inflammation will be managed and may even go away.

Clear any diet changes with your health care provider. You should stay on top of doing what you can for prevention and involving a professional in your care will help you to be healthier. If you suffer with health conditions that cause inflammation continue to follow your doctor's recommendations and protocol and add the dieting as a part of the treatment.

# Section 1: Anti Inflammatory Diet

An anti-inflammatory diet is highly recommended for those that have health problems, as food can cause inflammation that will make the problems worsen. The truth is that chronic inflammation is actually the cause of a number of diseases, such as cancer, Alzheimer's, and heart disorders. Avoiding foods that cause inflammation is important, but the many natural anti inflammatory foods that you can find in this book will help you to eat healthy and avoid inflammation. You'll find that you can protect your body easily, all by eating the right foods!

## Inflammation Problems

You notice swelling when it's on the outside of your body, such as when you injure yourself or you strain your muscles. You'll see the swelling, and it will cause you pain. You'll usually take steps to deal with that swelling, such as by applying ice or using heat to treat the problem.

When it's on the inside, it will take a lot more for you to

notice the swelling problems. You won't usually feel the inflammation unless it is very bad, and by then there's usually something seriously wrong. You'll have no idea if there isn't serious inflammation, at least not until your problem has gotten out of control. Whether it's swelling caused by arthritis, cancer, or heart disorders, you want to avoid that inflammation as much as possible.

# The Anti Inflammation Diet

The anti inflammation diet isn't a weight loss diet, but it's one that is designed to help you keep your inflammation under control. The anti inflammatory diet menu is filled with top anti inflammatory foods that will help to prevent swelling. Some of the best anti inflammatory foods include:

- **Fish --** Most fish contains Omega-3 fatty acids, which are excellent at fighting swelling. You'll find that salmon is one of the best foods to eat if you want to prevent swelling, making it top on the list of anti inflammatory foods.

- **Olive Oil --** Extra virgin olive oil should be included in all anti inflammatory diets, as the healthy unsaturated fats in the oil will help to fight off infection at its source. It will also protect your heart, so it's a healthy choice for anyone!

- **Kelp --** Kelp and other forms of seaweed are loaded with fiber, but it will also help to fight off swelling. It's rich in antioxidants, meaning that it will be a useful tool in the fight against cancer.

- **Blueberries --** These little berries are storehouses of nutrients, and they are known for being rich in antioxidants. They will help to fight off swelling, and they can help to prevent problems like dementia and cancer.

- **Crunchy Greens --** If it crunches and it's green, it's one of the best anti inflammatory diet foods for you to eat. Cruciferous vegetables contain more than just fiber, but they all have nutrients like antioxidants, folic acid, and vitamins to help prevent swelling.

- **Sweet Potatoes --** These tubers are one of the best natural anti inflammatory around, as they are loaded with the nutrients that your body needs to fight the swelling. These nutrients include beta-carotene, Vitamin B6, and manganese.

- **Garlic --** The aromatic cloves of garlic deserve their place in anti inflammatory diet recipes, as they're loaded with allicin, sulfur, and other minerals and antioxidants that are excellent at fighting swelling in your body.

- **Ginger and Turmeric --** These two spices are loaded with nutrients, and both of them will help to prevent swelling in the body.

- **Green Tea --** The antioxidants in the tea make this your beverage of choice for your anti inflammatory menu, and you'll find that there are many delicious ways that you can prepare this swelling-preventing tea!

What foods should you stay away from while on you anti inflammatory diet?

- Sugar, refined sugar, processed syrups, artificial sweetener. Use natural honey, molasses, and the natural sugar found in fruits to add sweetness to your food.

- Trans fats, saturated fats, cheap cooking oils, oils that have a high saturated fat content, peanut butter, margarine, most vegetable oils, and partially hydrogenated oil.

- **Alcohol.**

- Dairy products such as milk, sweetened yoghurts, full fat cheese, and cream. Some natural yoghurts are acceptable, and kefir is a good alternative.

- Meats from animals that are fed grain and corn, animals that have had fat injected, and red meat. You can eat very lean meat no more than once a week, but try and eat more poultry, fish, and legumes.

- White rice, white flour, noodles, pastries, baked

goods, and any refined grains.

- Artificial ingredients, with MSG and Aspartame being at the top of the list of foods to avoid.

- Foods that cause allergic reactions. If you are allergic to foods, the allergic reaction will include swelling, which can be fatal if the swelling occurs in your throat or lungs.

# Tips for Cooking and Eating Right When on the Anti Inflammatory Diet

If you're going to try the anti inflammatory diet and follow the list of anti inflammatory foods, it's important that you know how to cook. Eating right is more than just avoiding putting the wrong foods into your meals, but it's about know how to prepare the food. Here are some things you need to know about cooking and eating the right way while on the anti-inflammatory diet:

- **Make It Easy --** If you're going to be trying this diet, there are limits to what you can eat. You should try and make it as easy on yourself as possible, and you can do so by buying a variety of foods to prepare. Make sure that your diet has as much fresh food as possible, as that is the food that will be healthiest and reduce your risk of inflammation. Cut processed and artificial foods out of your diet, and make sure that you buy only the raw, healthy ingredients. Focus on eating more fruits and vegetables, and your diet will succeed!

- **How Many Calories? --** Do you know how many calories you need to eat in order to be healthy? The average adult male needs to consume about 2,400 calories per day, while the average female needs to consume more like 1,900. The smaller you are and the less activity you do, the fewer calories you need to eat. You shouldn't have to worry about gaining weight while on this diet if you eat right, so make it a habit to eat the right number of calories in your day. Make sure that you're getting carbs, protein, and healthy fats at each meal, and you shouldn't have to worry about inflammation!

- **Watch the Carbs --** Carbohydrates are both very important and very potentially dangerous. They are the nutrients that usually lead to inflammation, especially the simple carbs found in refined, white, sugary, and processed foods. Make sure that your diet includes no more than 200 to 300 grams of carbs per day, and try to make most of those carbs healthy complex carbs from whole grains, fruits, and veggies. Your food should all be low on the Glycemic Index, and should be as free of sugar and syrup as possible. You will be only eating foods that are whole or all-natural, but you still need to watch how many carbs you eat every day.

- **Be Careful with Fats --** Red meat contains fats, as do vegetable oils, dairy products, baked goods, and many other things that you're cutting out of your diet. However, remember that fat comes in all forms, so be careful even while on the anti inflammatory diet. Stay away from the oils that have high saturated fat content, and stick with the healthier oils like sesame, peanut, and olive oil. Make sure to eat lots of nuts, fish, and avocadoes -- all of which are loaded with healthy fats that will prevent inflammation. Remove the skin from any chicken or turkey that you eat, and find the meats that are as lean and fat-free as possible.

- **Protein is Important --** While on the anti-inflammatory diet, protein is one of the most important nutrients that you can eat. You're going to be cutting way back on carbs and fat, so you'll need to keep your body healthy by loading it with healthy proteins. Proteins like fish, tuna, and legumes are your best options, but chicken, turkey, and even lean meat can be part of your diet. You shouldn't eat more than 120 grams of protein per day, and make it lean and natural proteins as much as possible. Vegetable protein from beans and tofu are your best option to stay healthy while on this anti inflammatory diet.

- **Load the Fiber --** Seeing as you are trying to flush all of the inflammation-causing nutrients out of your body, it's in your best interest to speed up the flushing process. There are few nutrients that are as effective at getting rid of toxins and inflammation-causing chemicals as fiber, which comes from legumes, whole grains, and raw foods. Your best option is to eat as much of these foods as possible, as they will contain the nutrients that will keep your body healthy while you're trying to get rid of the unhealthy toxins and chemicals that are causing problems. You need to get at least 40 grams of fiber in your diet per day, so eat more fiber-rich foods while on the anti inflammatory diet for the best results!

- **Get Lots of Nutrients --** You need vitamins and minerals, as well as fatty acids and antioxidants. You can get these nutrients from all manner of places, though fruits and vegetables are some of the best sources. Carrots contain Vitamin A, citrus fruits contain Vitamin C, avocadoes contain Vitamin E, and berries, green tea, and red grapes contain healthy antioxidants. Make sure to get enough of the nutrients to stay healthy while on the anti inflammatory diet.

# Are You Cooking Right?

If you're cooking, you may be using more oil than you realize. If you're going to try this healthy diet, it's important that you cook the right way. Here are some cooking methods to stick with while on the anti inflammatory diet:

- **Poaching --** Cooking your food in water instead of oil may seem like a bad idea, but your food will come out just as tasty if you poach it correctly. You can use chicken broth to make the food taste better, and you'll find that soup base makes a great liquid for poaching. It will help your food to be healthier, and it will be equally delicious.

- **Baking --** Baking is the best way to keep your oil consumption limited. You don't actually need oil to bake food, but a bit of fat helps to keep the food tasty. Use olive or sesame oils for baking, and make sure that your food is in the center of the baking tray in order to enable air to circulate around the food. If you marinate the food before baking it, it will be juicy and moist. You can also use tin foil to cover the baked food, as it will trap the liquid inside the food.

- **Stir-Frying --** If you're going to cook your food with oil, you should use the stir-frying method made popular in China. The food doesn't sit in the oil - which stimulates the production of trans fats - but it will be just as tasty. The food doesn't absorb a lot of oil, and it will be much healthier.

- **Steaming** -- For vegetables, steaming is the best way to go. You won't have to do more than place the veggies in a steamer to get them to come out just right, and you can enjoy lightly-cooked veggies within minutes. Just make sure not to overcook them, as that will leech the nutrients out of the veggies.

- **Grilling/Broiling** --One of the best things about broiling and grilling your food is that it will not require any oil, but the natural juices in the food will make it tasty. Grilling is ideal if you have a grill, but a broiler is like a grill in the oven for those who don't have an easy-to-use grill. You will find far less fat in your food, and it will be a whole lot tastier!

It's very important that you avoid deep frying, frying, and microwaving your food. Boiling will leech the nutrients out of the food, unless you're making a soup that will utilize the water in which it was boiled. Make sure to cook the right way, and your food will be a whole lot healthier!

Now that you know what to eat and what not to eat - as well as how and how not to cook your food - you're ready to get started with the many recipes for your anti inflammatory diet!

Good luck, and happy eating!

# Delicious Anti Inflammatory Recipes

## Baked Teriyaki Chicken

This delicious dish will be perfect when served for dinner, and you'll find that it will be an absolutely delightful meal to enjoy any day of the week!

**Ingredients:**

For this dish, you will need:

Two chicken breasts
1 tablespoon of cornstarch
Water
Soy sauce
Orange juice
Rice or apple cider vinegar
Garlic
Fresh ginger root
Black pepper
1 cup of brown rice

**Preparation:**

To begin, chop two cloves of garlic into very small pieces, dicing it as finely as possible. Place a large skillet on the stove to heat, and pour a tablespoon of sesame oil into the pan. Once the sesame oil is hot, add the garlic into the bottom of the skillet, and cook for a minute - until the garlic begins to turn golden.

Drop the rice into the skillet, and cook the rice until it starts showing signs of toasting. Pour in 2 cups of water, and let it cook with the lid on. The rice will usually take about 35 minutes to cook properly, but check it occasionally to ensure that it doesn't burn.

As the rice is cooking, slice the chicken breast into four pieces. Rub the pieces of chicken breast with a little bit of salt and black pepper, and place them in a baking tray. Heat the oven to 350 F.

In a saucepan on the side, combine 3 tablespoons of orange juice with ½ cup of soy sauce and ¼ cup of vinegar. Apple cider vinegar will make the sauce a bit sweeter. Stir until the liquid is hot and nearly boiling, and drop the tablespoon of cornstarch into the pan. Stir for a minute, and turn off the heat.

Chop 4 cloves of garlic and about one tablespoon of fresh ginger root, and use the chopped aromatics to rub down the chicken once again. Pour the sauce over the chicken, ensuring that all of the breasts are covered equally.

Place the chicken in the oven, and let it cook for at least 15 minutes. Check to ensure that the chicken is properly cooked by inserting a knife. Make sure that the chicken is properly cooked, and that there is no raw meat in the center of the breast.

Serve the chicken on a bed of brown rice, and enjoy!

## Polynesian Chicken

This fascinating recipe combines savory chicken with sweet fruit, and it will be a unique dish that will make your mouth water.

**Ingredients:**

For this dish, you will need:

3 chicken legs and thighs
1 peach
¼ pineapple
1 bunch of grapes
Salt and pepper, to taste
Garlic
Sesame oil

**Preparation:**

To begin, remove the skin from the chicken. Cut the chicken in half, separating the legs from the thighs.

Turn the oven on, and let it heat to 350 F.

Dice the peach, pineapple, and grapes, and squeeze 1 orange and 1 lemon into the bowl of fruit to add some sweet flavor.

Dice the garlic very finely, and use it along with the salt and pepper to rub down the chicken. Add sesame oil to season the chicken, and place them in a baking tray. Top with the fruits, and place the chicken into the oven.

Give the chicken about 45 minutes to cook, as you will want to turn the heat down to about 325 F in order to avoid burning the fruits. Make sure the chicken is completely cooked by inserting a fork into the thickest part of the chicken, until it touches the bone. If no blood comes out, the chicken is properly cooked.

Remove the chicken from the oven, and transfer it onto a plate. Serve with barley, couscous, quinoa, or brown rice.

## Turkey Tenderloins

If you just can't stand the thought of spending all day preparing Christmas dinner, this is a quick and easy meal that you can make that will be just as tasty!

**Ingredients:**

For this dish, you will need:

2 pounds of turkey tenderloins
Soy sauce
Dijon mustard
Rosemary
Salt and pepper, to taste
Garlic
Onions

**Preparation:**

To begin, place the turkey tenderloin in sealable plastic bags.

In a bowl, combine ½ cup of soy sauce with 2 tablespoons of Dijon mustard and 4 teaspoons of crushed rosemary. Add salt and pepper as desired, and mix thoroughly. Dice the onions and garlic as finely as possible, or run them through a food processor before adding them into the mixture.

Once the sauce is properly mixed, pour some of the sauce into each bag. Shake the bag well to ensure that the liquid has coated the turkey tenderloins completely, and place the bags in the fridge.

The turkey should sit in the fridge for at least 3 or 4 hours, as that will ensure that the meat has absorbed the flavor of your marinade. You may want to give the bags a shake every hour, as that will ensure that both sides are coated with the liquid.

Preheat the oven to 350 F when you are ready to cook the turkeys. Remove the turkey tenderloins from their bags, and place them in an oven tray or broiler pan - depending on your desired doneness of the turkey. Let them broil or bake for about 25 minutes, checking to ensure that the turkey is properly cooked. Poke it with a knife to check for doneness, and the turkey will be properly cooked when the juices run clear.

Slice the turkey, and serve with the rest of your dinner.

## Turkey Curry

This fantastic dish will enable you to use all those leftovers from Christmas dinner, or you can use ground turkey if you want a delicious variation on a traditional Indian dish. It may be a bit spicy, but it's guaranteed to be absolutely delightful!

### Ingredients:

For this dish, you will need:

Sesame oil
Ground cinnamon
1 onion
4 cloves of garlic
Fresh ginger root
Turmeric root
Water
2 green chili peppers
1 pound of turkey meat (ground or diced turkey)
Red chili powder
Garam masala
Salt and black pepper, to taste
2 cups of brown rice

**Preparation:**

To begin, place the rice in a skillet to cook. You will need about 2 cups of water per cup of brown rice, but add an extra half cup to ensure that the rice doesn't turn out crunchy once it's done cooking. Place a lid on the rice, and leave it to cook for about 40 minutes.

Place another skillet on the stove to heat, and add in 2 tablespoons of sesame oil into the pan. Add half a teaspoon of cinnamon into the pan, and mix it in with the oil. When the oil gets hot, the cinnamon's scent will be released.

When you can smell the cinnamon, add the diced onions into the pan. Cook them until they are golden brown, and add the garlic in to cook for about a minute. Dice 1 tablespoon of ginger root and 1 teaspoon of turmeric root, and add them into the pan to cook with the garlic. The ginger and turmeric should cook for about three minutes in order to release all of their flavors into the food.

Once the aromatics have cooked, add ¼ cup of water into the pan. Bring the water to a boil, and let it thicken the roots. Cut the two green chilies in half, and add them into the pan. Add the turkey, a teaspoon of spicy chili powder, and ½ teaspoon of garam masala. Add another half cup of water, and place a lid on the curry as it cooks.

You will want to let the curry cook for about 10 more minutes, as that will ensure that the turkey is properly cooked. Once the mixture has thickened into a sauce, add a bit of salt and pepper for flavor. Taste the sauce, and add water to thicken it if necessary.

Serve over the brown rice, and enjoy!

## Noodle-Free Turkey Lasagna

This dish will be the perfect addition to your anti inflammatory diet menu. You'll be able to enjoy the classic taste of the dish, but without having to worry about noodles, red meat, and ricotta cheese causing swelling in your body. It tastes great, but it's a lot lighter than your average lasagna.

**Ingredients:**

For this dish, you will need:

1 pound of ground turkey
8 large tomatoes
1 onion
5 cloves of garlic
Basil
Thyme
Oregano
6 ounces of Cottage cheese
4 zucchini
Salt and pepper, to taste

**Preparation:**

To begin, cut the onion in half, and add half into a pot -

along with 3 cloves of garlic. Cut the tomatoes in half, and place them in the pot to stew. The tomatoes will need to cook for about an hour, as that will soften them and make it easier to run them through your food processor.

Puree the tomatoes after an hour of cooking, and place them back into the pot to continue cooking. Add in salt and black pepper, as well as a teaspoon of fresh basil, a pinch of thyme, and a teaspoon of oregano. Stir the sauce well, and let it cook for another hour. (Add water as needed as the liquid boils down).

Once the sauce has cooked properly, remove it from the stove. Dice the other half of the onion and the two remaining garlic cloves, and place them in a skillet with a tablespoon of olive oil. Cook the aromatics until they are golden brown, and add the ground turkey into the skillet to cook. Make sure that the ground turkey has been cooked properly, and remove the skillet from the stove.

Add a bit of salt, pepper, garlic, and oregano into the cottage cheese, and use the cottage cheese. Slice the zucchini into thin strips, and place them in a baking tray - as you would lay out regular lasagna noodles.

Pour tomato sauce onto the zucchini, and scoop the

ground turkey onto the first layer. Cover with a layer of zucchini, more tomato sauce, and the cottage cheese. Continue adding layers until the tray is full, and the ingredients are all used up.

Preheat the oven to 350 F, and place the trays in the oven to bake. It will take about 20 minutes for the zucchini to cook, and you can remove the trays from the oven and serve while the lasagna is still hot!

## Black Bean Huevos Rancheros

This Mexican recipe is the perfect breakfast, and you'll find that the delicious addition of black beans makes it a very healthy meal that will be surprisingly filling!

**Ingredients:**

For this dish, you will need:

4 eggs
2 tomatoes
1 onion
1 green chili pepper
1 cup of canned black beans
¼ pound of turkey or soy bacon
Salt and pepper, to taste

**Preparation:**

To begin, dice the bacon into small pieces. Place a skillet on the stove to heat, and fry the bacon in the bottom of the pan. Once the bacon is becoming crispy, add the black beans into the mix. Cook the beans until the liquid is boiling and the beans are hot.

In a separate pan, add a tablespoon of olive oil, and

place the pan on the stove to heat. As the pan is heating, dice the onion very finely. Add the onion into the pan, and cook until golden brown.

While the onions are cooking, dice the tomatoes into small cubes. Add them into the pan, and let them cook for about 5 minutes. Add salt and black pepper, as desired.

Dice the chili pepper into very small pieces, and add it into the pan with the other ingredients. Let the chili cook until it is soft, and remove the ingredients from the pan. Return it to the stove, and add a tablespoon of olive oil once again as the pan heats.

Crack the eggs into a bowl, and beat the eggs thoroughly to combine the yolks and the whites. Pour the eggs into the pan, and cook them as scrambled eggs. Once they are properly cooked, add the tomato mixture and the black beans into the dish. Mix the eggs together with the other ingredients well, and serve with some brown flour tortillas and homemade salsa!

## Quinoa Breakfast Cereal

Need a healthy, hot breakfast to get your day started off on the right foot? This delicious breakfast cereal is made with quinoa -- a low-glycemic grain that will not cause inflammation in your body. Add to that the high fiber of prunes, and you've got a breakfast for champions!

**Ingredients:**

For this dish, you will need:

Water
1 cup of quinoa
1 cup of prunes
1 cup of almond milk
Cinnamon
Nutmeg
Salt

**Preparation:**

To begin, place the quinoa in a saucepan to cook, along with a cup of water. Once the water is boiling, cover the quinoa and let it cook for about 5 more minutes - or until the grains are fairly soft. The total cooking time for the quinoa will be under 15 minutes, so keep a close eye on it.

Once the quinoa is cooked, pour in a cup of almond milk and keep the fire on low. Add in a pinch of salt, and half a teaspoon each of nutmeg and cinnamon. Remove the pits from the prunes, and add them into the quinoa to cook.

You will be able to eat the breakfast cereal once the prunes have softened, and enjoy the delicious way to start your day!

## Hearty Bean Dinner

This is a wonderful dish to make on a budget, and you'll find that it will be a filling meal that will be surprisingly cheap. If you want to save money and still eat well, this is definitely the dish you should try!

**Ingredients:**

For this dish, you will need:

2 cups of dried beans
Water
1 onion
1 clove of garlic
1 stalk of celery
1 potato
3 tomatoes
½ pound of soy or turkey bacon
1 tablespoon of honey
1 bunch of cilantro
Salt
Mustard powder
Oregano
Black pepper, to taste

**Preparation:**

To begin, place the dried beans in a large pot to cook, and add about 4 cups of water for every cup of beans. Drop the onion, the head of garlic, the celery stalk, and the potato into the water -- leaving them whole and unpeeled.

Set the pot on the stove to cook, and let the beans boil for about 3 hours. You'll want to add a bit of salt into the beans as they cook, and let them cook until the skin of the beans will crack when you blow on them.

Once the beans have cooked properly, use a ladle to fish out the onion, garlic, potato, and celery. Throw these into the garbage, as they will have absorbed all of the gas from the beans -- but will have released their flavors into the legumes.

Dice the tomatoes into cubes, and add them into the beans. Pour 3 cups of hot water into the beans, along with a tablespoon of salt and black pepper each. Place the beans back on the stove, and let them cook.

As the beans continue cooking, place a skillet on the stove for the bacon. Cook the bacon in the pan until it is golden brown, and add it into the beans -- along with any oil that is produced by the bacon.

Add the cilantro into the pot, and use a teaspoon of mustard powder and oregano each to add flavor to the beans. Let them cook until you can smell the variety of flavors, and let the beans boil for a few minutes to ensure that they absorb all of the delicious tastes.

Serve while hot.

## Quinoa and Black Beans

If you want a healthy, low fat meal to enjoy while on your anti inflammatory diet, this is definitely a dish for you to enjoy! It will have almost no effect on your blood sugar levels, as both quinoa and black beans are low GL foods. It is a delicious meal that will fill you up easily and quickly!

**Ingredients:**

For this dish, you will need:

Sesame oil
1 onion
5 cloves of garlic
1 cup of quinoa
Cumin
Cayenne pepper
Salt and pepper
2 ears of corn
1 can of black beans
Fresh cilantro

**Preparation:**

To begin, place the quinoa in a pot with water, and place

the pot on the stove to cook. You'll need about a cup of water per cup of quinoa, but add a bit extra water just to be safe. The quinoa will take about 15 minutes to cook on medium heat, so keep a close eye on it.

Place the ears of corn in a pot, and add enough water to cover the corn. Bring the pot to a boil, and cook until the corn is soft. Remove the corn from the pot, run them under cold water to cool them down, and use a knife to remove the kernels of corn from the cob. Place the corn kernels in a bowl and set them aside.

Place a skillet on the stove to heat, and add a tablespoon of olive oil into the pan. Dice the onion and garlic very finely, and add them into the stove to cook as well. Cook them until they are golden brown, and add the quinoa into the pan to cook as well. Mix the quinoa well to ensure that the flavors of the garlic and onions are absorbed into the grain.

Once the quinoa has been stirred into the aromatics well, add a teaspoon of cumin and ½ teaspoon of cayenne pepper. Add the black beans and the ears of corn, as well as half a bunch of cilantro -- chopped before adding, of course.

Mix the ingredients together well, let them cook for a

few more minutes, and serve while hot.

## Meaty Beans and Rice

This dish is guaranteed to have your kids begging for more, even if beans aren't their favorite food. It's a recipe that's quick and easy to make, and you'll find that the dish will be a popular one with your whole family.

**Ingredients:**

For this dish, you will need:

1 pound of ground turkey or chicken
1 cup of dried beans
2 onions
1 head of garlic, plus 5 cloves
1 potato
3 tomatoes
Tabasco sauce
Brown Rice
Water
Cumin
Crushed red pepper
Oregano
Salt and pepper, to taste

**Preparation:**

To begin, place the beans in a pot with 4 cups of water per cup of beans. Place the pot on the stove to heat, and drop 1 whole onion, 1 head of garlic, and the whole potato into the beans. This will absorb the gas, and will add the flavor into the beans.

Let the beans cook for about four hours, or until blowing on the beans will cause the skin to crack. Once they are cooked, use a ladle to scoop out the onion, garlic, and potatoes, drain the water from the beans, and return them to the stove with three cups of water added to the pot.

Dice the tomatoes into small cubes, and add them into the pot of beans. Dice half of the other onion, as well as three cloves of garlic. Add them into the pot, and let the beans cook for about half an hour more.

As the beans are cooking, place the brown rice in a pot on the stove to cook, using about 1 cup of brown rice and 2 ½ cups of water. Bring the brown rice to a boil on high heat, and turn the fire to low heat to let the rice cook until it is soft. Add more water as needed to prevent the rice from burning.

Place a skillet on the stove to heat, along with a tablespoon of olive oil. Dice the two remaining cloves of garlic, along with the remaining half onion. Cook them until they are golden brown, and add the ground meat into the pan. Brown the meat before adding a tablespoon of crushed red pepper, a teaspoon of cumin, and a teaspoon of oregano. Add salt and pepper as desired. Finish cooking the meat, and remove from the stove.

The beans should be cooked by now, so remove them from the pot they are in and pour them into a skillet on the stove. Pour in half a cup of almond milk, as well as salt and black pepper. Use a masher to mash the beans, making sure that 90% of the beans are properly mashed.

Pour the refried beans into the pan with the meat, and mix them well before serving over a bed of brown rice.

## Lentil Soup

If you are feeling chilled on a cold winter day, there's nothing like a hot bowl of soup to help you warm up! This delicious soup contains all of the nutrients you need to stay healthy, and you'll find that it will be the perfect meal to eat when the weather turns chilly.

**Ingredients:**

For this dish, you will need:

1 cup of lentils
Olive oil
1 onion
4 cloves of garlic
2 carrots
2 celery stalks
4 large tomatoes
Salt
Black pepper
Bay leaves
Water
Fresh parsley
Paprika

**Preparation:**

To begin, place the lentils in a bowl, and fill the bowl with drinking water. Leave the lentils to soak in the water overnight, as that will help them to cook a lot faster - and will eliminate the gas from the legumes.

Come the next day, drain the lentils, run water over them again to rinse them out, and drain them thoroughly.

Place a soup pot on the stove, along with a couple of tablespoons of olive oil. Dice the garlic very fine, and add it into the pot. As the garlic is cooking, dice the onions to be added once the garlic has turned slightly golden. Dice the celery stalks as well, and add them once the onions have become partially translucent. Add the carrots in next, and stir fry everything in the soup pot for a few minutes.

Before you add in the lentils, drop a teaspoon of paprika, a couple of bay leaves, a tablespoon of salt, and as much pepper as you want into the onions. Sauté everything together for a few minutes, and finally add in the lentils.

Add enough water to cover the lentils completely,

working with about 4 cups of water per cup of lentils. Bring the water and lentils to a boil. Dice the tomatoes into small cubes, and add them into the boiling soup. The water will cook the tomatoes quickly, and turn it into a delicious soup. Don't forget to add the parsley before removing the soup from the stove and serving while hot.

## Chicken and Lentils

If you want a unique dish that will make your mouth water and your stomach rumble, this is the one for you. You'll find that it takes a bit of work to make, but it's absolutely fantastic and an excellent choice for any occasion!

**Ingredients:**

For this dish, you will need:
Olive oil
2 large chicken breasts
1 onion
3 carrots
4 cloves of garlic
1 cup of lentils
Salt
Cilantro
4 tomatoes
Rosemary
Basil
Thyme
1 lemon
Black pepper, as desired

**Preparation:**

To begin, place the lentils in a mixing bowl, and fill the bowl with water. Leave the lentils to soak overnight, as that will eliminate the gas and make the lentils easier to cook. The following morning, drain the lentils, rinse them well, and drain them once again before setting them aside.

Place a skillet on the stove, and add a few tablespoons of olive oil into the bottom of the pan. Slice the chicken breast from the bone, and cut each breast into three pieces. Cook the pieces in the skillet, making sure that the breast is properly cooked before removing it from the fire.

Heat the skillet once again with oil, and dice the onion to add into the pan. Cook until tender, and add the diced garlic into the pan. Dice the carrot as well, and add it into the pan to cook for about 5 minutes.

Cut the tomatoes into cubes, and bring them to a boil on the stove. Cook them until they are nice and saucy, and they will turn into a thick tomato sauce.

Once the carrots have cooked, transport the aromatics into a soup pot, heat the pot, and add the lentils into the pot. Mix them around to coat them with the flavor and the oil from the aromatics, and pour 3 cups of water into the pot. Add as much salt as you want, and let the lentils cook for about 20 minutes once the water has begun to boil.

Place the chicken back in the used skillet, and continue cooking on low heat for a few more minutes. Transport the chicken into the pot with the lentils once they're cooked, and stir well to ensure the chicken is coated with the flavor.

Add the tomato sauce into the pot, as well as a teaspoon each of basil and rosemary. Let the lentils keep cooking with these added ingredients for another 5 minutes or so, and serve with a dash of lemon juice for flavor.

## Curried Lentils

Nothing makes a good curry like some lentils mixed with chicken, and you'll find that this exotic dish will be just what you need to help you fill up on a healthy meal. With the addition of brown rice or quinoa to the mix, you can make a healthy, filling dinner!

**Ingredients:**

For this dish, you will need:
½ cup of lentils
1 can of unsweetened coconut milk
Curry paste
Salt
Water
2 chicken breasts
Quinoa
8 cloves of garlic
1 onion

**Preparation:**

To begin, place the lentils in a bowl, and fill the bowl with water. Place the bowl in the sink, and let the lentils soak overnight. This will make them easier to cook the next day, and will eliminate a lot of the gas. Come morning, drain the lentils, rinse them, drain them again, and set them aside.

Place the lentils in a sauce pan, and add a cup of water into the pan. Turn the heat to high, and bring the lentils to a boil. Once they are boiling, add a tablespoon of curry paste and the coconut milk. Stir well to ensure that the ingredients are mixed, and add a pinch of salt. Cover the curry with a lid, and turn the heat on low to allow the lentils to simmer gently.

In a separate skillet, add a tablespoon of olive oil. Dice 5 cloves of garlic and ¾ of the onion, and sauté them in the bottom of the skillet.

Cut the chicken breasts into small cubes, and cook them in the skillet with the aromatics. Once the chicken is nearly cooked, add it into the curry mixture and mix well. Return the lid and let the lentils continue cooking.

Place the skillet back on the stove to heat, and add a tablespoon of olive oil. Dice the remaining garlic cloves and the rest of the onion, and sauté them in the bottom of the pan. Add 1 cup of quinoa, and cook until the quinoa shows signs of becoming toasted. Add 1 ½ cups of water, and turn the heat down to medium to allow the quinoa to cook. It will take about 15 on medium heat, so make sure to watch the quinoa.

Once the quinoa is cooked, serve it onto a plate, and scoop the curried lentils on top. Add a dash of lemon for flavor, and garnish with a sprig of parsley or cilantro.

## Maple-Flavored Salmon

If you're a fish lover, salmon is the best of the best! You'll find that the rich taste makes it incomparable, and the fatty acids in the fish make it excellent for preventing inflammation. This recipe will help you to make a fish that you just can't help but love!

**Ingredients:**

For this dish, you will need:

1 pound of salmon fillets
¼ cup of natural maple syrup (not the artificially produced kind)
Soy sauce
4 cloves of garlic
Salt
Black pepper
Fresh ginger root
1 lemon

**Preparation:**

To begin, combine the maple syrup in a bowl with about half a cup of soy sauce. Add in a pinch of black pepper, half a tablespoon of salt, and the minced garlic. Add half a tablespoon of chopped fresh ginger root, and a dash of lemon. Stir well to combine all of the ingredients.

Place the salmon fillets in a baking tray with a bit of olive or sesame oil coating the bottom of the tray. Preheat the oven to 350 F.

Pour the sauce over the fish fillets, and set the tray in the fridge to marinade while the oven is heating. Once the oven is hot, place the baking trays in the oven, and let the salmon cook without a cover for about 20 minutes.

The salmon will be ready to eat once it flakes when you press on it with a fork.

## Grilled Salmon

If you're a fan of grilled fish, this is a recipe that you can't help but love! You'll find that it's absolutely fantastic when you make it on a wood-fire grill, but you can cook it up on the stove or a propane grill if you want. It will be just as tasty, and a lot less work to prepare!

**Ingredients:**

For this dish, you will need:

1 pound of salmon
Balsamic vinegar
1 lemon
Soy sauce
Salt
½ an orange
Fresh ginger root
Paprika
Black pepper
Red pepper flakes
5 cloves of garlic
3 green onions
Sesame oil
Peanut oil

**Preparation:**

To begin, slice the salmon into steaks. It will be easier to marinade and rub the fish if it's already sliced up.

In a bowl, combine ¼ cup each of soy sauce and balsamic vinegar with the juice from one large lemon. Add in the juice from the orange, and dice or grind the garlic and ginger very finely to add them into the mix. Add in a teaspoon each of black and crushed red pepper, paprika, and sesame oil, and as much salt as you think it needs. Dice the green onions, and add them into the mixture. Stir well to combine.

Pour the sauce over the fish, and use your hands you rub the various ingredients into the fish gently. Add a bit of peanut oil, and transfer the salmon fillets into Ziploc plastic bags. Pour the sauce into the bags, and shake to coat the fish with the liquid completely. Set the steaks in the fridge to marinade, and let them sit for about an hour as you fire up the grill.

You want the heat of the grill to be medium high, so either turn down the propane grill or wait until your wood fire has mostly burned down to red coals. Remove the salmon fillets from their bags, place them on the grill, and cook them until they are tender and flaky. Use a brush to apply some of the liquid, and they will taste heavenly once you're done!

## Baked Garlic Salmon

This is a delicious fish dish that you can't help but love, and you'll enjoy the rich flavor of this amazing salmon. Even those that aren't partial to fish will find this recipe entirely enjoyable, and it's one of the best anti inflammatory recipes that you can prepare!

**Ingredients:**

For this dish, you will need:
1 pound of salmon
4 cloves of garlic
Fresh dill
1 lemon
3 green onions
Salt and pepper, as desired

**Preparation:**

To begin, turn the oven to 425 F, and let it heat as you go about preparing the fish.

Slice the salmon into steaks, ensuring that they're neither too thick nor too thin. Spray some cooking spray on aluminum foil, and place the salmon steaks onto the foil.

Sprinkle a bit of salt and black pepper onto the fish, as your taste demands. Dice the garlic and the onions very fine, and add a bit of the aromatics into the foil with the fish. Slice the lemon, and place one or two thin slices on each piece of fish. Add the fresh dill -- chopped, of course -- as the final touch.

Once the fish has been seasoned, use a piece of tin foil to cover the top of the fish - wrapping it tightly to ensure that the juices will not leak out. Place the wrapped fish steaks in a baking tray, and place the tray in the oven.

The salmon should take about 20 to 30 minutes to cook, and you can check to see that the salmon is done by pressing on the steaks with a fork. If it flakes easily, they're ready to eat.

## Salmon Ceviche

This recipe comes from South America, specifically Peru - the land of the Incas. It's a unique dish that will surprise you, and it's an absolutely fantastic one when it's made right.

**Ingredients:**

For this dish, you will need:

1 pound of sushi-grade salmon (it is fresh enough to eat raw)
¼ tablespoon of natural brown sugar
Salt
Chili sauce
3 Limes
Black pepper
Cumin
Olive oil
2 cloves of garlic
1 small red onion
1 tomato
Fresh cilantro
1 avocado

**Preparation:**

To begin, add the brown sugar into a bowl with ½ teaspoon of chili sauce and 2 tablespoons of salt. Stir well, adding the juice from the three limes into the bowl. Add ¼ teaspoon each of cumin and black pepper, along with the same amount of olive oil.

Dice the garlic and the onion very fine, and stir them into the bowl. Dice the tomatoes and the cilantro, and add them into the mix. Cut the salmon into bite-sized cubes, and stir the salmon gently into the other ingredients.

The salmon will need to sit in the fridge overnight, though you can eat it after about 4 to 6 hours. Drain the liquid from the salmon, cut the avocado into cubes, add the cubes into the mix, and serve the delicious fish dish cold with whole wheat crackers.

## Mixed Veggie Salad

If you want to keep cool during the summer, this delicious salad will definitely be the ideal dish for you! It will be a refreshing veggie dish that will go well with any meal, or you can even make a hearty main dish out of it by adding fish or chicken.

**Ingredients:**

For this dish, you will need:
1 head of lettuce
1 tomato
1 red onion
1 ear of corn
1 cucumber
1 head of cabbage
1 bunch of spinach

**Preparation:**

To begin, place the spinach and lettuce in a bowl to soak. Make sure to wash the spinach well, as you want to get all of the dirt out from among the leaves.

Dice the tomato into cubes, and place them in a bowl. Slice the onion into rings, and add them into the bowl as well.

Place a stock pot on the stove to heat, and add the ear of corn into the pot with 2 cups of water. Bring the water to a boil, and cook the corn until you're sure that it's properly tender. Use a knife to cut the kernels from the ear, and add the kernels into the salad.

Slice the cabbage very finely, and do the same for the lettuce. Cut the spinach into thin strips, and add the three leafy vegetables into the salad.

Cut the cucumber in half, and scoop out the majority of the slightly bitter seeds from inside. Slice the cucumber into small pieces, and add them into the salad. Toss the salad well, and add the dressing of your choice for a refreshing mixed vegetable delight!

## Grilled Chicken Cranberry Spinach Salad

If you want a hearty salad that will be very filling, this is the one for you for! You'll be able to get all of the nutrients that you need, and without eating any simple carbs or refined foods. Just from the salad, you'll be filling your body with all the healthy nutrients that will keep it running!

**Ingredients:**

For this dish, you will need:

1 large chicken breast
1 bunch of spinach
½ cup of cranberries
½ cup of nuts (pecans, almonds, etc.)
¼ cup of poppy seeds
½ red onion
¼ cup of white wine vinegar
¼ cup of apple cider vinegar
¼ cup of peanut or olive oil
Salt and black pepper, to taste

**Preparation:**

To begin, slice the chicken breast into medium sized

pieces. You should get about 12 pieces from the chicken breast.

Place a skillet on the stove, and cook the chicken with a tablespoon of olive oil in the bottom of the pan. Make sure that the chicken's juices run clear, and remove them from the pan to cool in a plate on the side.

Slice the spinach, or use your hands to rip it apart. Add the cranberries, nuts, and poppy seeds into the bowl, and toss the salad.

Dice the red onion very finely, or run it through your blender. Mix the vinegars and the oil together, and use them to dress the salad. Toss the salad gently, and top with the grilled chicken breast.

## Delicious Cucumber Salad

This salad will be an absolute delight, and you'll find that it will be one of the most enjoyable salads that you can eat while on the anti inflammatory diet. It's easy to make, and it requires very few ingredients to prepare.

**Ingredients:**

For this dish, you will need:

2 cucumbers
3 tomatoes
1 red onion
Mayonnaise
White vinegar
Salt and black pepper, to taste
Dill

**Preparation:**

To begin, slice the cucumbers in half. Cut the halved cucumbers into slivers, making sure that they are thin enough to eat easily. (Note: The peel on some cucumbers will be very bitter, so peel them if necessary.) Cut the tomatoes into slivers as well, and add them into the bowl with the cucumbers. Cut the onion into thin rings, and stir them in with the cucumbers.

In a separate bowl, combine 3 tablespoons of vinegar with a tablespoon of white vinegar. Add salt and pepper as desired, and mix the dressing in with the vegetables.

## Tofu Salad

If you're a tofu lover, this is definitely the salad for you! It's loaded with all the healthy nutrients your body needs, and you'll find that it will be a surprisingly filling side dish despite the fact that it's mostly made with vegetables.

**Ingredients:**

For this dish, you will need:
1 package of firm Tofu
Korean sweet chili sauce
Ginger root
2 cloves of garlic
Soy sauce
Sesame oil
1 cup of snow peas
2 carrots
1 head of red cabbage
1 cup of peanuts

**Preparation:**

To begin, combine the chili sauce with a tablespoon each of soy sauce and sesame oil in a bowl. Dice the garlic until it's very fine, and crush the ginger. Add both of the aromatics into the sauce, and stir well. Cut the tofu into cubes, and add it into the sauce. Place the mixture into the fridge, and let it marinate in the cool fridge for about an hour.

Place a pot of water on the stove to heat, and leave the pot on high heat until the water is boiling. Turn the water to medium heat, and drop the snow peas into the water. Let them sit for about 3 minutes, and scoop them out with a slotted spoon. Place them in a bowl of cold water to cool off for a few minutes, and drain them before setting them aside.

Slice the cabbage very finely, and use the grater to grate the carrots into long, thin strips. Chop the peanuts as much as you can.

Add the carrots into the bowl with the cabbage, and add the snow peas as well. Toss the vegetables to mix them, and add the dressing with the tofu to complete the flavor. Garnish the salad with peanuts, and serve.

## Tofu Scramble

If scrambled eggs in the morning aren't your thing, you may find that this delicious tofu scramble will be your best option! It's a vegetarian's dream, and it's a delightfully low fat meal that you can enjoy at any time of the day!

### Ingredients:

For this dish, you will need:
1 pack of firm silken tofu
Olive oil
1 onion
4 cloves of garlic
1 green bell pepper
2 potatoes
2 green tomatoes
Salt

### Preparation:

To begin, peel the potatoes and cut them into bite-sized pieces. Place them in a pot on the stove, along with enough water to cover the potatoes. Turn the heat on high, and bring the potatoes to a boil. Cook them until they are just soft enough to spear them with a fork, and remove them from the heat.

In a skillet, place a tablespoon of olive oil. Dice the garlic very fine, and add it into the bottom of the skillet. Once the garlic has turned slightly golden brown, add the potatoes into the skillet. Cook them until the potatoes are properly tender, and remove them from the pan.

Place the skillet back on the stove, along with two tablespoons of olive oil. Dice the onions as the oil is heating, and add them into the skillet to cook. Once the onion has become tender and slightly transparent, add the green bell pepper -- which you will have de-seeded and diced. Cook until the bell pepper is soft.

Dice the green tomatoes, and add them into the skillet. Cook them until they begin to release their juices, and add the salt as desired. Add the potatoes into the mix, and cook for a few more minutes.

Once the potatoes are properly coated with the juices of the tomatoes, add the tofu into the pan. You will need to mash it using a masher or a fork, as that will make it much easier for you to scramble. Mix the tofu in with the rest of the ingredients, and let it cook until it gets nice and hot.

Serve with bran muffins or whole wheat toast

## Baked Tofu

This is a dish that you'd never expect to enjoy, but it's surprisingly enjoyable! Even if you aren't a tofu enthusiast, it's very likely that you'll love the taste of this dish. It may take time to get used to, but it's a healthy meal that will grow on you with time.

**Ingredients:**

For this dish, you will need:
1 pack of firm tofu
Soy sauce
Sesame seeds
Ginger
Honey
1 cup of brown rice
Water

**Preparation:**

The night before you are going to eat the dish, crush the ginger and add it into a bowl with 3 tablespoons of soy sauce. Remove the tofu from the package, and drain it thoroughly before putting it into a Ziploc plastic bag. Pour the soy sauce mixture into the bag, and shake it to coat the tofu. Place it in the fridge to marinate overnight. In the morning, turn the tofu over to allow the other side to marinate properly.

Place the brown rice in a pot with 2 ½ cups of water, and cover the rice with a lid once the water has begun to boil. It will take the rice about 45 minutes to cook completely, and you may have to add a bit more water to ensure that it doesn't burn.

As the rice is cooking, toast the sesame seeds in a pan. Keep the fire on low heat, and add about ½ cup of the seeds into the pan once it is already hot. It will take about three minutes to toast the seeds.

Once the seeds have been toasted, let them cool off on a plate, and sprinkle the cool seeds onto the tofu once you have removed it from the plastic bag. Preheat the oven to about 350 F, and place the tofu into the oven to bake for about 8 minutes once it has heated properly. Make sure to pour the remaining marinade over the tofu, and serve the baked tofu on a bed of rice -- sprinkled with the rest of the seeds.

## Lime and Cilantro Tofu

This is a unique Tofu-rich twist on a classic Latin American dish, and you'll find that it has all the great taste that you've come to expect from Mexican and South American food. It's a rich dish that will set your mouth watering immediately.

### Ingredients:

For this dish, you will need:
1 pack of extra firm tofu
Cilantro
4 cloves of garlic
2 limes
Soy sauce
Cumin
Natural brown sugar
Cayenne pepper
Olive oil

### Preparation:

To begin, dice fresh cilantro until you have about a handful of the green stuff - or ¼ cup. Dice the garlic very finely, and add it into a bowl with the cilantro. Grate the zest from the 2 limes, and add it into the bowl with the garlic. Squeeze the lemon juice, and add it into the bowl as well. Add in a teaspoon and a half of soy sauce, a teaspoon of the cumin, half a teaspoon of brown sugar, and half a teaspoon of cayenne pepper. Pour in about a tablespoon of olive oil, and mix all of the ingredients together well.

Open the package of tofu, drain the liquid, and add the large cube of extra firm tofu into a Ziploc plastic bag. Pour the marinade into the bag, and shake the tofu gently to coat it with the liquid. Once it has been properly coated, place it in the fridge to marinate. You can leave it overnight if you want, or it will be good to eat in about an hour.

Once the marinating is done, remove the tofu from the bag - using a slotted spoon to allow the liquid to drain off the tofu.

Place a skillet on the stove to heat, and add a tablespoon of olive oil into the bottom of the pan. Place the marinated tofu in the skillet, and cook it until it has been evenly browned on all sides. Apply the marinade each time you flip the tofu, and that will ensure that it absorbs all of the delicious flavor. It will take about 15 minutes to cook, and you can serve the cooked tofu on a bed of brown rice.

## Tofu Watercress Salad

This delicious salad will be the perfect side dish for a hearty meal, or it will help you to stay faithful to your diet. It's a very low fat and low calorie dish, but it's loaded with the healthy nutrients that your body needs!

**Ingredients:**

For this dish, you will need:
Bean sprouts
1 pack of firm tofu
2 cans of tuna
2 tomatoes
1 bunch of watercress
Pickled radish
½ red onion
4 cloves of garlic
Sesame oil
Soy sauce

**Preparation:**

To begin, pull out a baking dish to prepare the salad in. Cover the bottom of the tray with bean sprouts, and follow it with a layer of tofu. Drain the tofu and slice it into thin pieces to lay on top of the bean sprouts. Open the cans of tuna, drain the liquid, and layer the tuna on top of the tofu.

Cut the watercress into strips, and add a layer on top of the tuna. Dice the tomatoes into small cubes, and use them to make the next layer of the salad. The top layer will be the Japanese pickled radish, and you can use as much of that as you like.

Dice the onion very fine, and place it in a bowl. Place a skillet on the stove to heat, and add a tablespoon of sesame oil into the bottom. Dice the garlic, and add it into the skillet to cook. Make sure the garlic has browned properly, and use a spoon to scoop the garlic pieces from the skillet. Add the onions into the skillet to cook, and cook them until they too are browned.

Add the garlic pieces into the salad on top of the radish, and cover the salad with the sesame oil and the cooked onions. Add half a cup of soy sauce into the salad, and stir it well to mix everything together. Serve with crackers, or as a standalone dish.

## Fruit Salad

This delicious fruit salad will get your body going in the morning, or it will be the perfect dessert to enjoy after a hearty meal. The best thing about it is that it's 100% natural and healthy, so you can have it anytime and anywhere!

**Ingredients:**

For this dish, you will need:
Strawberries
1 red apple
1 green apple
Berries (blueberries, raspberries, etc.)
2 kiwi fruits
½ pineapple
Grapes

**Preparation:**

To begin, cut the stalk from the top of the strawberries. Cut the strawberries in half, and add them into a bowl.

Cut the red apple in half, and use your knife to remove the core. Cut the halves into thirds, and cut each of the resulting slices into bite-sized pieces. Repeat the same process with the green apple.

Place the berries into a colander, and run cold water over them. Raspberries can be damaged if the pressure of the water from the sink is too high, so make sure the water is gentle.

Cut the core out of the pineapple, and cut the rest into slices. Each round slice can be cut into eight pieces, and add the pieces into the bowl with the strawberries, apples, and berries.

Peel the kiwi fruit with a paring knife, and cut the ends off of the fruit. Cut the kiwi into slices, and cut each slice into quarters before adding them into the bowl.

Run the grapes under cold water, and drain them thoroughly. Cut them in half, and add the halves of the grapes into the bowl with the rest of the fruits.

Garnish with a bit of wheat germ, a sprinkling of natural brown sugar, and enjoy!

## Healthy Oatmeal

If you want to start the day out with a meal that will be very enjoyable as well as filling, this is the breakfast for you. It's quick and easy to make, and you'll have no problem eating it while on the anti inflammatory diet!

**Ingredients:**

For this dish, you will need:

1 cup of steel cut oats
3 cups of water
1 cup of almond milk
½ cup of assorted nuts
½ cup of raisins and cranberries
Flaked coconut
Cinnamon
Vanilla
Honey

**Preparation:**

To begin, place a pot on the stove, and add the three cups of water into the pot. Add a pinch of salt, and bring the water to a rolling boil. Once the water has begun to boil, drop the oats into the water. Cook them for about

20 minutes, or until soft. (The steel cut oats will get soft very quickly, so keep an eye on them.)
Once the oats have cooked properly, remove them from the fire. Add the milk into the oats, and stir in the cranberries and raisins.

Use a knife to chop the nuts, and add them into the oats as well. Add a tablespoon of the flaked coconuts, and stir 2 teaspoons of vanilla extract into the oatmeal. Add two tablespoons of honey to make the oatmeal sweet, and add a pinch or two of cinnamon.

Return the pot with the oatmeal to the fire, and turn the fire on low. You will need to stir the oatmeal continuously, mixing the oats with the milk and the other ingredients. Don't let the oatmeal burn, but just leave it on the stove long enough to heat up the oatmeal once the oats have been added.

Serve with a sprinkling of wheat germ, sesame seeds, and amaranth seeds to make your oatmeal healthy and filling!

## Banana Nut Breakfast Cereal

This is a meal that is guaranteed to keep you healthy, and you'll find that it's one of the tastiest breakfasts that you can eat. It will be loaded with nutrients, and you will definitely enjoy it once you get used to its unique, varied flavor.

**Ingredients:**

For this dish, you will need:

Water
1 cup of almond milk
Quinoa
1 banana
Oats
Oat bran
Cinnamon
Salt, for flavor
Assorted nuts
Brown sugar
Vanilla extract

**Preparation:**

To begin, place a sauce pan on the stove to heat. Add a

tablespoon of quinoa into the pan, along with ½ a cup of almond milk and a few tablespoons of water. Once the mixture has begun to boil, turn the heat down to its lowest setting.

Let the oatmeal mixture simmer for about 5 minutes, and test frequently to ensure that the quinoa is getting soft. Once the quinoa is soft, add the banana into the pan. Use a fork to mash it, and stir it in with the quinoa.

As the banana is cooking with the quinoa, add a tablespoon each of oats and oat bran. The mixture should get thicker very quickly, and it's the sign that the ingredients are cooking properly. You will need to keep it cooking on very low heat for about 5 more minutes, though stir it gently to ensure that it doesn't burn.

Once the mixture has thickened, add a tablespoon of brown sugar, a teaspoon of vanilla extract, and a pinch of salt and cinnamon each. Chop the walnuts into small pieces, and add them into the cereal to give it the delicious nutty flavor that makes it the perfect breakfast!

All of these recipes can be found online, though some of them are our own original creations. You can probably find similar recipes on websites like AllRecpes.com,

About.com, and particularly ElanasPantry.com. They are all recipes that someone made, and we just wanted to share them with you. We've made a few adjustments to the various recipes so that you'll get only our unique grain-free flavor on the recipes, but you'll find that there are many like them. The important thing is that you can enjoy your grain-free cooking and eating, and we wanted to provide you with a recipe book that you can use to prepare delicious meals free of grain and gluten. We apologize if you've seen these recipes elsewhere, and we hope that you enjoy the creations we have presented to you!

# Section 2: Grain Free Cooking

Grain free eating can be hard to think about in a culture that uses flour, corn and other refined starches in almost every food. For some of us, however, grains aren't the healthiest option. Mounting evidence suggests that heavy carbohydrate consumption simply isn't ideal for a significant portion of the population. If you're among these people, you're better off choosing a protein-heavy diet that helps you keep your blood sugar consistent and reduces your risk of diabetes and similar conditions.

For others, the gluten found in a wide variety of grains like wheat, rye and some oats can cause serious digestive and metabolic problems. Whether you have a grain allergy or you suffer from gluten intolerances such as celiac disease, your body simply can't digest grains properly. In severe cases, the nutritional deficiencies caused by this problem can lead to fuzzy thinking, deterioration of the bones and teeth, and even serious mood disorders. The solution is simple: just discontinue grains.

Last but not least, you may wish to avoid grains if you're following a paleo-style diet. These eating plans focus on the foods that were available to our ancestors before the advent of agriculture. That means that grains were consumed infrequently at best, and they were never processed into flour or other highly refined products. The diet relies much more heavily on fresh fruits, vegetables, tubers and animal products such as meat. If you follow a paleo diet, you'll find plenty of material here to keep your taste buds happy and your body healthy.

# The Problem of Grains

Grains such as wheat, rice, corn, barley and rye have been an essential part of human diets all over the world since the invention of agriculture. They are appealing, easy to produce in large quantities, and simple to cook. Unfortunately, they aren't necessarily the ideal option for many people. Modern varieties of grains may be especially prone to problems. They have been modified extensively from their ancestral form, containing far more starch and less fiber than their ancestors. In many cases, they seem to be more likely to cause metabolic diseases, intolerances and other problems than even the grains that were available just a century ago.

The problem becomes even more serious when genetically-modified foods appear on the scene. While the basic mechanism of genetic modification is the same whether the process occurs in the field through breeding or in a lab, modern science makes gene tinkering extremely easy. We don't know whether this process has any significant side effects, however. Since many of the grains currently on the market have been genetically modified, it can be hard to tell whether they're having an effect on your health.

These issues are part of why so many people are choosing to limit or eliminate grains in their diet. While grain free dieting isn't for everyone, a significant percentage of the people who try it find themselves feeling stronger, more energetic and healthier. Headaches, excess weight gain and even some long-lasting health problems decrease and even vanish in many people. In many cases, it seems as though our bodies simply aren't meant to use grains in the forms that are currently available.

# Transitioning to a Grain Free Diet

If you have reason to believe that you could benefit from a grain free diet, you may still have trouble making the leap. After all, most cultures still have a basic diet that is built on one or more grains. Whether it's the ubiquitous bread found in North American and European cooking, the corn we see in so much native and Central American cuisine, or the rice found throughout Asia, grains seem to be everywhere. By choosing to eliminate them from your diet, you have to deliberately go against the flow. Many people who are seeking to cut out excess grain consumption have run into trouble finding good, healthy recipes to help them.

The key is to approach the process carefully and with a well-defined plan. If you're hoping to cut your carbohydrates or want to use a paleo-inspired diet plan, you may want to slowly substitute more grain free foods in your diet. Over time, you can replace your favorites with foods that are just as delicious, without seriously disrupting your life.

For others this method won't work as well. This is the

case if you know you have a serious allergy or intolerance to one or more grains. You may also have trouble with the slow substitution technique if you are using specific kinds of low carbohydrate diets. In these cases, you'll need to start over from scratch. Remove all the grain based foods from your home and avoid picking up new ones to reduce temptation.

No matter how you make the transition, it's important to have a plan. Haphazardly trying to start on a new way of eating is one of the surest ways to guarantee the failure of this lifestyle change. Instead, make sure you have a good idea of what's available to you in your new, grain-free lifestyle, and choose the most appealing foods you possibly can. It's much easier to make the switch when you know that you have something to look forward to.

# A Question of Nutritional Balance

If you're like many people, you're probably used to getting the bulk of your nutrition from grain-based foods such as bread or pasta. That can make transitioning to a diet that's lower in or completely free of grains a little daunting. After all, no one wants to discover that they've been eating a nutritionally imbalanced diet after making this kind of change, and many government health organizations recommend eating up to 11 servings of grains every day.

In reality, consuming this many grain-based products isn't necessary for good health. Many cultures consume far less, basing their diets on non-grain starches, fresh fruits and vegetables, and healthy meats with no significant health issues. As long as you pay attention to the basic recommendations of your specific grain-free diet plan or your nutritionist, you shouldn't have too many problems with balance. Focus on eating a variety of different foods instead of just the same few every day, and you'll soon be feeling healthier and happier than you ever did while consuming lots of processed grains.

# Grain Free Shopping and Cooking Tips

Shopping for grain-free foods can be extremely difficult, especially if you're used to consuming a lot of convenience foods. That's because many apparently non-grain products actually contain extremely processed grain ingredients. For instance, many ketchups, pasta sauces and even commercial French fries have been treated with dextrose, glucose and maltodextrin. These sweeteners are derived from corn or rice, and they can be incompatible with a non-grain diet.

You may also find grains in non-dairy milks, baking powder, spice mixes, flavored beverages and many other foods. If you choose any kind of prepared meat, such as pre-made hamburger patties, there is a good chance that a corn, wheat, or rice-based thickener and binder has been used in its preparation. Even soy sauce usually contains hidden wheat unless otherwise labeled. Read packages carefully and avoid any product that contains thickeners, malt ingredients, dextrose and similar sweeteners, non-specific starches such as modified food starch, or ingredients labeled simply as "vegetable" or "plant" proteins.

It's also important to be careful in the kitchen, especially if you suffer from an allergy or intolerance. In shared cooking spaces, it's very easy for grains from a roommate or family member's cooking to end up in your food. Wash all knives, cutting boards, counters and containers carefully before using them to reduce the risk of contamination. While this may not be a concern for everyone, in some cases even a small amount of a grain-based product can make you very sick.

# Reading the Recipe Key

Since there are so many reasons to seek out grain free recipes, not every meal will be right for every kind of diet. This book uses the symbols **GF**, **P** and **LC** to mark gluten-free, paleo and low carbohydrate recipes to ensure that you can quickly and easily find the perfect dish for your next meal. While most recipes will meet the requirements of more than one type of diet, it's important to check before you start cooking if you want to ensure perfect nutrition for your dietary requirements.

# Breakfast

## No-Grain Granola (GF, P, LC)

Breakfast cereal is an important part of many people's regular daily routine, but it can be hard to have cereal without grains. This no-grain granola recipe relies on fresh raw nuts and seeds rather than oats or wheat. It's sweetened naturally with dates and uses no oil, so it's suitable for all kinds of low-carbohydrate diets. You'll enjoy this rich, delicious and very natural breakfast option, whether you have it with fresh fruit and your favorite dairy or plant milk or you eat it on its own. To increase the sweetness, just add more date paste.

**Ingredients**

2 cups raw pecans
2 cups raw cashews or Brazil nuts
2 cups raw pumpkin or sunflower seeds
1 cup plain coconut flakes
1 cup dates
1 cup water
½ cup flax seeds
1 vanilla bean or 2 teaspoons vanilla extract
½ teaspoon cinnamon or mixed sweet spices

Place the whole nuts and seeds in a large bowl and cover them with lukewarm water, stirring to combine. Allow to rest at room temperature for 8 hours to 2 days. This process sprouts the seeds and removes phytic acid, which can cause digestive problems. In a food processor or blender, combine the dates and 1 cup of warm to hot water. Process for about 1 minute, or until a smooth paste is formed. Split the vanilla bean and scrape out the contents.

Drain the nuts and seeds, then add the coconut flakes,

flax seeds, vanilla, date paste, vanilla scrapings and cinnamon. Stir to combine. Line a baking sheet with parchment paper and pour the granola mixture out onto it, spreading into an even layer. Dehydrate in 170 degree Fahrenheit oven for about 8 hours or until the granola is crunchy. Stir periodically to break up clumps. Allow to cool and place in an airtight container for storage. This mixture lasts for 3 to 4 weeks at room temperature.

## Fresh Homestyle Beef Sausages (GF, P, LC)

Most commercial sausage recipes rely on grains as fillers and binders for the meat. This makes the sausage easier to prepare and protects the manufacturer's bottom line, but it can be disaster for your grain-free diet. Making your own sausage at home is a surprisingly simple way to enjoy this classic breakfast meat without worrying about the inclusion of oatmeal, wheat, pork or other undesirable substances. For a different flavor, substitute chicken.

### Ingredients

2 pounds grass-fed boneless chuck steak
1 tablespoon fresh thyme
1 tablespoon fresh sage
¾ tablespoon coarse salt
½ teaspoon red pepper or sharp paprika

Trim the fat from the meat and discard, then chop the beef into cubes approximately 1 inch across. Freeze on a baking sheet for about 20 minutes, or until the texture is relatively firm. Combine the herbs, pepper or paprika and salt in a small bowl. Remove the meat from the freezer. Place ½ of it in the refrigerator and place the other half in the bowl of a powerful food processor.

Sprinkle with about ½ of the spice mixture and pulse until the meat is in very small pieces and the spices are well incorporated throughout.

Spread a piece of parchment paper on a counter or cutting board and transfer the meat to the center of the paper. Roll the paper around the meat to form a log, twisting the ends to secure them or using a rubber band. Repeat the process with the remaining meat and spices to form two fat sausages. Freeze for 30 minutes before cooking to make the slicing process easier. Cook in ¼ inch thick slices over medium-high heat and serve with eggs, sauces, soup or on pizzas. This recipe can be frozen for up to 2 months without loss of flavor.

## Almond Cottage Cheese Pancakes (GF, P*, LC**)

Pancakes and other breakfast sweets can be hard to come by when you're on a grain-free diet, but that doesn't mean you have to give them up completely. This recipe uses starches derived from tubers, not grains, along with flour from nuts and seeds. If you've been missing that classic pancake breakfast, this is the recipe for you.

**Ingredients**

½ cup almond flour
½ cup cottage cheese
3 large eggs
1/8 cup coconut flour
1 tablespoon raw honey
3/8 teaspoon baking powder
¼ teaspoon cream of tartar or lemon juice
¼ teaspoon plain gelatin granules
¼ teaspoon vanilla extract
salt to taste
2 tablespoons coconut oil

Place the almond flour, cottage cheese, eggs, coconut flour, honey, baking powder, cream of tartar, gelatin, vanilla and salt in a food processor or blender and process until combined and completely smooth. Heat 1 tablespoon of coconut oil in a heavy-bottomed skillet or griddle to medium-high. Spoon the batter into the pan in a thin layer about 4 inches across and cook until the bottom is golden and the top looks relatively dry. Flip and cook until the other side has browned. Remove the cakes from the pan and repeat until all batter has been consumed. Serve with fruit, yogurt, honey, syrup or jam.

*This recipe is not suitable for paleo dieters who avoid dairy products or eggs.

** To make this recipe low-carbohydrate friendly, omit the honey or substitute a no-calorie liquid sweetener according to package instructions.

## Open-faced Apple, Egg and Salmon Sandwich (GF, P, LC)

This breakfast recipe combines the richness of egg with the sharp sweetness of a tart baking apple and the salty savor of salmon. Look for organic apples whenever possible. This recipe makes four sandwiches, but it's easy to cut back to serve just one or two.

6 large eggs
4 slices smoked salmon
2 large tart baking apples, such as Granny Smith
2 tablespoons coconut oil
salt and pepper to taste
Romano cheese (optional)

Crack the eggs into a medium bowl and beat until thick and creamy. Season with salt and pepper. In a medium pan, heat the coconut oil to medium-low. Pour in the eggs and allow to set, then scramble, cooking for about 5 minutes. Remove from heat. Core the apples and slice each one in half. Place the apple halves cut-side-up in an oven-safe baking dish. Top each piece of apple with a slice of salmon and ¼ of the scrambled eggs. Garnish with thinly-shaved Romano cheese if desired. Bake at 400 degrees Fahrenheit for 10 minutes, or until apples are warm throughout.

## Almond Waffles (GF, P*)

Using almond flour produces a crunchy waffle that makes an excellent snack. Make sure that you preheat the waffle iron for at least 15 minutes before cooking this recipe, since a cold iron can result in trouble removing the finished waffles. Serve with fresh fruit, coconut oil or butter, cream or maple syrup.

**Ingredients**

2 ¾ cup almond flour
2 ¾ cups tapioca flour
2 3/4 cups water
1/4 teaspoon salt
1 tablespoon coconut oil

Brush the waffle iron with coconut oil and preheat. Combine the almond flour, tapioca flour and salt in a large bowl. Add the oil and water, stirring vigorously until well combined. Allow the batter to stand for five minutes, then remix before pouring the individual waffles. Pour about 1 ½ cups of batter into the waffle iron at a time and cook on high heat for 15 minutes or until the surface is crisp and golden. Reheat the waffle iron and re-stir the batter before cooking each set of waffles.

* Some paleo diets permit the use of starch from tubers such as tapioca or arrowroot, but this may not apply to all cases.

## Green Eggs (GF, P, LC)

With or without the addition of your favorite non-pork "ham," this recipe will definitely turn heads and please your taste buds. The addition of flavorful, nutrient-dense fresh kale makes simple scrambled eggs bright green and highly unusual. For a change, consider substituting parsley or spinach instead of the kale.

### Ingredients

4 large eggs
½ pound kale
coconut oil for frying
salt and black pepper to taste

Remove the ribs and stems from the kale and discard. Combine the remaining leaves with the eggs, salt and pepper in a blender and process until completely smooth. Heat the oil to high in a large skillet. Pour the egg mixture into the pan and allow it to set, then scramble gently with a silicone spatula or wooden spoon until creamy and cooked through. Serve with breakfast sausage or your favorite non-grain bread.

## Hot Porridge (GF, P, LC)

Hot porridges such as oatmeal may not be romantic, but many people find that they miss these foods' simple appeal when it's time to give up grains. This comforting version is based on nuts and seeds, but it still has that creamy texture. For a savory version, substitute black pepper for the cinnamon and serve with butter, paprika, cheese or even crispy bits of turkey bacon.

### Ingredients

1 cup water
¼ cup chopped walnuts
2 tablespoons plain shredded coconut
1 tablespoon pumpkin or sunflower seeds
1 tablespoon chia seeds
1 tablespoon flax seeds
1 teaspoon cinnamon
¼ teaspoon salt

Bring the water to a boil. Combine all the other ingredients in a powerful blender and process until a fine meal is produced. Pour the boiling water over the entire mixture and cover. Blend slowly, increasing the intensity, until the porridge is smooth and creamy. Serve hot, with dried fruit, cream, honey or milk.

## No-Grain Breakfast Burritos (GF, P, LC)

Breakfast burritos are a tasty and convenient way to enjoy a savory start to your day. When corn and wheat tortillas are no longer an option, we turn to egg tortillas instead. Filled with taco meat, guacamole and other tasty ingredients, this also makes an excellent light lunch.

### Ingredients

1 pound ground turkey
2 ripe avocados
1 small red onion
1 medium tomato
1 lime
2 cloves garlic
2 tablespoons cilantro
1 teaspoon salt
1 tablespoon grain-free taco seasoning
12 eggs
1 tablespoon grain-free hot sauce
1 tablespoon coconut oil.

In a skillet over medium heat, brown the turkey. Sprinkle the meat with 1 tablespoon of taco seasoning, stirring to combine. Remove from heat. Mash the avocados, chop the onion, tomato, cilantro and garlic, and combine in a small bowl. Season with salt and lime juice, mixing until you have achieved your preferred consistency.

In a separate skillet, heat the coconut oil to medium-low. Beat two eggs until creamy and thick. Season with salt and hot sauce, then pour a thin layer into the hot skillet. Allow to cook all the way through on one side and remove to a plate. Repeat the process until you have 12 egg tortillas. To serve, top each tortilla with a spoonful of taco meat and guacamole. Garnish with green onions or sour cream if desired.

## Sweet Potato Breakfast Casserole (GF, P, LC)

This quiche-like dish uses grated sweet potatoes to produce an appealing and grain-free crust, into which are piled eggs, meat, cheese and fresh herbs. Substitute your favorites to produce variations on this exciting brunch casserole. This dish is great hot and fresh out of the oven, but it can also be served cold for lunch or a snack.

### Ingredients

2 medium sweet potatoes
4 eggs
¾ cup diced turkey or your favorite breakfast sausage
2 tablespoons coconut oil
1 small onion
1 tablespoon fresh basil
1 tablespoon fresh oregano
1 tablespoon flat-leaf parsley
Salt to taste
½ cup cheddar cheese (optional)

Grate the sweet potatoes finely. Grease a pie plate using 1 teaspoon of coconut oil. Salt the sweet potatoes and press them evenly over the sides and bottom of the pan. Melt the coconut oil and pour it over the layered sweet potatoes. Bake in a 425 degree Fahrenheit oven for 20 minutes, or until crisp but not burnt. Remove and allow to cool slightly.

Spread turkey or sausage in an even layer over the bottom of the crust. Sprinkle cheese over the meat. In a small bowl, beat the eggs thoroughly. Chop the herbs and add them to the eggs. Season with salt to taste and pour over the meat and cheese. Reduce the oven temperature to 350 degrees and bake for 30 minutes or until the center is solid. Allow to set slightly, slice and serve.

# Main Dishes

## Pot Roast with Fresh Vegetables (GF, P, LC)

A traditional pot roast makes a great addition to almost any grain-free dinner. About half the fat in the beef is monounsaturated, or “good” fat. Plus, this meat is full of vitamin B12 and other essential nutrients. When combined with mustard, garlic and other delicious spices, it's an easy and appealing choice for just about any meal. It also freezes well, making this roast a good option for single-serving meals later.

### Ingredients

5 pounds chuck roast
2 pounds mushrooms
2 large onions
1 ½ pounds carrots
4 cups butternut squash
2 cups beef broth
2 tablespoons tomato paste
2 tablespoons sunflower oil
1 small head garlic
1 tablespoon thyme

1 tablespoon sharp paprika
1 teaspoon salt
1 teaspoon black pepper
2 bay leaves

Trim the excess fat from the roast. In a small bowl, combine the salt, mustard, thyme, pepper and paprika. Rub this mixture over the outside of the roast. Heat the oil in a large Dutch oven to medium-high. Place the roast inside and brown on all sides, turning periodically. Peel and coarsely chop the onions and garlic. Add these to the pot along with the stock and tomato paste. Bring all to a simmer and cover, cooking for about 10 minutes.

Remove from heat and place the entire pot in the oven. Bake at 325 degrees Fahrenheit for 3 hours. Coarsely chop the mushrooms, carrots and squash. Remove the roast and add the vegetables, then recover and bake for an additional hour. Serve immediately right from the pot.

## Tropical Tilapia (GF, P)

Once unknown, tilapia has become one of the most common whitefish options. This species has tender flesh with a mild flavor, plus it's harvested from fish that repopulate readily and live in a wide range of environments. That makes it a better choice than many traditional whitefish, whose numbers are on the decline. Originally from tropical habitats, tilapia taste delicious when combined with other hot-climate foods such as pineapple, coconut and sweet potatoes.

### Ingredients

1 pound tilapia fillets
2 large sweet potatoes
1 large onion
2 cups coconut milk
1 tablespoon coconut oil
¼ cup fresh pineapple
salt and black pepper to taste

Bake, boil or steam the sweet potatoes until they are tender and remove the skins. Slice them into thick rounds. Heat a tablespoon of coconut oil in a large frying pan over medium heat. Dice the onions and cook them in the oil until they are softened and translucent, but not brown. Stir the coconut milk to emulsify any solids and add it directly to the onions. Bring to a simmer, then add the tilapia fillets in a single layer. Cook the fish in the coconut milk mixture for about 5 minutes or until the bottom side is opaque. Flip the fillets and add the pineapple in a single layer on top. Cook the entire pan for an additional five minutes, then serve on top of the sweet potato rounds. Drizzle the remaining coconut milk and onion mixture on top of the dish and season with salt and pepper.

## Barbecue Chicken with Grain-free Sauce (GF, P)

Barbecue lovers are often disappointed when they go grain free, since most commercial barbecue sauce is chock full of ingredients derived from wheat, rice and corn. Fortunately, it's extremely easy to make your own delicious barbecue sauce at home. These very simple chicken wings are excellent hot or cold, and they make the perfect addition to just about any cookout.

20 chicken wings
1 cup tomato sauce
1 large juice orange
3 shallots
½ cup honey
¼ cup vinegar
2 cloves garlic
1-inch piece ginger
1 teaspoon fresh thyme
1 teaspoon salt
½ teaspoon sharp paprika

Dice the shallots, garlic and ginger finely. Combine with all ingredients other than chicken wings in a medium-sized pan and simmer over medium-low heat until the onions are soft, or about 45 minutes. Allow to cool. Wash the chicken wings and remove the tips. In a large bowl, toss the wings with ½ cup of barbecue sauce. Place them in a 9 x 13 inch casserole pan and bake at 350 degrees Fahrenheit for 30 to 45 minutes. Use the shorter time period if you intend to finish the wings on a charcoal or gas grill. Otherwise, finish by turning the oven to broil and cook for approximately 10 minutes, or until wings are properly browned. Transfer to a large bowl and toss with another ½ cup barbecue sauce, then serve.

## Zucchini Pasta with Roasted Sweet Potatoes and Coconut Pesto (GF, P)

While meat makes up a big part of most grain-free diets, that doesn't mean it has to appear in every meal. This pasta-style squash dish is light and delicious, with a rich pesto-based sauce and plenty of protein from coconut. It also includes sweet potatoes to help ensure that it's filling as well as tasty. Unlike many of the recipes in this book, this zucchini pasta is best eaten fresh and does not store well.

### Ingredients

2 large zucchinis
2 medium sweet potatoes
1 cup mixed greens
1 cup fresh basil
½ cup plain shredded coconut
½ cup hot water
¼ cup olive oil
1 lemon
salt and black pepper to taste

Cut the zucchini into long ribbons using a spiral slicer or a paring knife. Chop the sweet potatoes into large pieces and toss with 1 tablespoon olive oil. Place in an oven-safe dish and roast at 375 degrees until tender. Set aside and allow to cool. Bring a pot of water to a boil over medium-high heat and add the zucchini. Cook for 2 to 3 minutes, or until zucchini is translucent but not mushy. Remove from water and plunge immediately into a bowl of ice water. Drain and set aside.

Juice the lemon. Combine in a blender or food processor with coconut, hot water, olive oil and basil. Season with salt and pepper to taste. Process until smooth and toss with finished zucchini pasta. Serve over salad greens, topped with sweet potatoes.

## American Taco Pie (GF, P, LC)

This Americanized Mexican dish is hearty and savory. It also freezes well in individual portions, making it an excellent choice for lunches or dinners on the go. Choose relatively lean ground beef, grass-fed if possible, for the best flavor.

### Ingredients

1 ½ cups almond flour
¼ cup coconut oil
1 teaspoon salt
1 pound ground beef
1 tablespoon olive oil
1 medium onion
1 sweet red bell pepper
1 avocado
2 tablespoons grain-free taco seasoning
salt and pepper to taste

In a large bowl, mix the salt, coconut oil and almond flour, blending until a moldable dough forms. Transfer this dough to a standard pie plate and press into an even layer over the whole surface. In a large skillet, heat the olive oil to medium-high. Chop the onions and cook until softened and translucent. Add the ground beef and brown until completely cooked. Mix in the taco seasoning, salt and pepper. Cook for an addition two minutes and remove from heat. Pour the beef mixture into the pie plate and bake for 30 minutes at 350 degrees Fahrenheit, or until the crust is firm. Chop the lettuce, pepper and avocado roughly. Top the finished pie with vegetables and serve immediately.

## Braised Chicken with Sweet Potatoes and Fennel Bulb (GF, P)

Chicken legs are inexpensive and flavorful, especially when combined with vitamin A-rich sweet potatoes and the unique taste of fennel. Don't be afraid of the amount of lemon juice required in this recipe; it helps brighten all the other tastes and adds a delightful natural tang that you shouldn't miss. For an extra touch, serve the chicken with a small curl of lemon peel as garnish.

4 chicken legs
2 cups chicken broth
3 medium sweet potatoes
1 bulb fennel
4 scallions
1 small head garlic
2 lemons
2 tablespoons coconut oil
salt and pepper to taste

Heat the coconut oil to medium high in a large skillet. Sear the chicken legs for about 5 minutes per side, or until lightly browned. Transfer to a large, oven-safe pot. Thinly slice the fennel and scallions. Mince the garlic and roughly chop the sweet potatoes. Reheat the skillet and add the fennel, cooking for about 5 minutes, or until the fennel is golden brown. Add the garlic and green onions, reduce heat, and cook for an additional 3 minutes or until the onions are wilted. Transfer the contents of the pan to the pot with the chicken. Juice the lemons and add the juice to the pot, along with the stock, salt and pepper. Cover and bake for 40 minutes at 300 degrees Fahrenheit, or until the chicken is cooked through and the sweet potatoes are tender.

## Baked Cashew Chicken (GF, P, LC)

This Asian-inspired main dish is rich, sweet and flavorful. It also provides plenty of manganese, magnesium and copper, essential nutrients that many people lack. This meal is great if you need extra energy or you're cooking for a big group. Because of the fat in the cashews and coconut milk, this dish may separate when chilled. Just warm it up again and stir to restore the texture.

### Ingredients

1 pound boneless, skinless chicken breast
2 cups water
1 cup cashews
½ cup coconut milk
¼ cup fresh mint
1 medium yellow onion
4 cloves garlic
1 lime
1-inch piece fresh ginger
2 tablespoons coconut oil
1 tablespoon ground coriander
1 tablespoon ground cumin seeds
1 teaspoon cinnamon
1 teaspoon cloves
salt and pepper to taste

Cut the onions into quarters and combine in a food processor with the cashews, ginger and garlic. Process until a soft puree forms and set aside. Heat the coconut oil in a medium pan over medium-high heat. Add the puree and stir-fry for about 5 minutes or until browned. Add the cumin, cloves, cinnamon and coriander and allow to cook for an additional 5 minutes, stirring periodically. Add the coconut milk and water. Season with salt and black pepper according to preference. Place the chicken in an oven-safe casserole dish and pour the coconut milk mixture over the meat. Cook at 300 degrees Fahrenheit for about 30 minutes, or until the chicken is cooked through. Serve with chopped mint and lime slices.

## Savory Braised Duck (GF, P, LC)

Most people eat plenty of chicken and turkey, but very little duck. In fact, some have never enjoy this rich, flavorful bird! This simple braised recipe makes it easy to enjoy the nutrient-rich dark meat of this slightly unusual type of poultry. If duck is unavailable, you can substitute chicken thighs or similar cuts, but duck is definitely best. Allow the dish to rest for a little while after cooking to produce the tastiest finished product.

### Ingredients

4 duck legs
1 cup duck or chicken stock
1 small head garlic
1 medium onion
1 stalk celery
2 medium carrots
1 ½ pounds tomatoes
1 small head broccoli
2 tablespoons flat-leaf parsley
1 tablespoon duck fat or coconut milk
1 tablespoon fresh thyme
salt and pepper to taste

Heat the duck fat or coconut oil in a large Dutch oven

over medium-high heat. Brown the duck legs, turning several times. Remove and set aside. Dice the garlic, onion, celery, carrots and tomatoes. Reheat the Dutch oven and sauté the vegetables in the remaining fat for about 5 minutes, or until tender. Return the duck legs to the pot and add the stock and thyme. Cook for approximately 90 minutes at about 325 degrees Fahrenheit, or until the carrots are soft and the duck is cooked through. Add the broccoli 15 minutes before the cooking process is done. Allow the meat to rest for 10 minutes, then serve garnished with parsley.

## Stuffed Bell Peppers with Veal (GF, P, LC)

Ordinary stuffed peppers rely on conventionally-grown hamburger, but this version uses tender veal for a different taste and texture. To get the best results, look for pastured veal rather than crate-raised, since the texture of the meat is much better. Despite the lack of carbohydrates, this meal is extremely filling. Consider packing an extra pepper or two for lunch the next day!

### Ingredients

1 pound ground veal
3 sweet red bell peppers
2 sweet orange bell peppers
3 tablespoons olive oil
1 medium red onion
½ pound cherry tomatoes
1 tablespoon fresh cilantro
1 tablespoon fresh oregano
1 tablespoon fresh marjoram
3 cloves garlic
salt and black pepper to taste

Remove the stems, ribs and seeds from all the bell peppers. Mince one red bell pepper and set aside. Cut the other four peppers in half, wash thoroughly, and arrange on a cooking dish, cut-side up. Brush with 1 tablespoon of olive oil and bake in a 350 degree oven for 20 minutes. Remove and set aside to cool.

In a separate pan, heat the remaining two tablespoons of olive oil to medium-high. Mince the garlic and onions and add to the pan, along with the minced red bell pepper. Saute for 2 minutes or until soft. Add the veal and season to taste using salt and black pepper. Cook, stirring occasionally, until the meat is done through. Add the fresh herbs and cherry tomatoes and continue cooking for an additional 2 minutes.

Stuff each pepper half with the meat mixture. Cover the entire pan with a sheet of aluminum foil or a lid and bake again for 25 minutes. Uncover and finish in the oven for an additional 10 minutes. Serve with a fresh salad.

## No-Rice Pad Thai (GF, P, LC)

Pad Thai, the famous stir-fried noodle dish, is traditionally made with highly-refined rice noodles. This version uses mung bean noodles, which lack some of the health problems normally associated with rice. For a version that's lower in carbohydrates, consider substituting Japanese Shirataki noodles, which are made from a yam-like tuber and are about 97 percent water. While the basic recipe is vegetarian, it's easy to add in your favorite meat or seafood for a heartier version.

### Ingredients

6 ounces dried mung bean noodles
1 large head broccoli
2 large onion
¼ cup peanuts or cashews
3 tablespoons coconut oil
4 scallions
3 cloves garlic
1 tablespoon sesame oil
1 tablespoon honey
1 teaspoon tamarind paste
1 teaspoon wheat-free tamari or fish sauce

Fill a large pot with water and bring to a boil over high

heat. Cook noodles according to package instructions, drain, and set aside. In a large wok or skillet heat the coconut oil to medium-high. Slice the onion, scallions and garlic. Stir fry the onion until lightly browned. Add the broccoli, breaking it up into individual florets. Stir fry until the broccoli turns bright green and becomes tender. Stir in garlic, followed by noodles. In a small bowl, combine sesame oil, tamarind paste, tamari and honey. Pour this mixture over the noodles and vegetable, stirring vigorously to prevent sticking and burning. Serve on individual plates garnished with scallions and crushed peanuts.

# Baking and Desserts

## Almond-coconut Chocolate Chip Cookies (GF, P)

Commercial chocolate chip cookies are loaded with preservatives, white flour, processed sugar and fillers. Even the kind you normally make at home require a number of heavily-processed, genetically modified ingredients. Skip those unappealing cookies in favor of this recipe, which relies on natural sugars, almond flour and coconut flour to provide plenty of nutrition without the starch. Stick to store-bought almond flour to ensure proper lightness; the homemade variety can yield a very flat cookie.

### Ingredients

5/8 cup almond flour
5 tablespoons unsalted butter
4 ounces grain-free dark chocolate
2 tablespoons honey or maple syrup
1 tablespoon coconut flour
1 large egg
1/3 teaspoon salt
¼ teaspoon vanilla extract

¼ teaspoon plain gelatin granules
¼ teaspoon baking soda

Bring butter to room temperature and combine with honey or syrup in a large bowl. Add gelatin, egg and vanilla. Allow the mixture to rest for 5 minutes. In a separate bowl, combine the almond and coconut flours, salt and baking soda. Add the dry ingredients to the wet mixture slowly, stirring continuously. Beat until combined. Chop chocolate into small pieces and stir into the cookie mixture. Line a baking pan with parchment paper. Scoop by teaspoonful's onto the pan, leaving plenty of space for the cookies to spread. Bake in a 350 degree Fahrenheit oven for 12 minutes, or until the edges brown slightly. Eat warm with a glass of your favorite dairy or plant milk.

## Honey-Buttermilk Panna Cotta (GF, P*, LC**)

Traditional panna cotta is naturally grain free, making it a great substitute for commercial puddings laden with corn starch. This version uses buttermilk for extra flavor and natural maple sweeteners. Whenever possible, stick to using real vanilla beans, which provide a more subtle and interesting taste than extracts. Enjoy this rich and appealing recipe with plenty of fresh raspberries or strawberries.

1 ½ cups natural buttermilk
1 cup heavy cream
1/3 cup maple syrup
1 tablespoon warm water
2 ¼ teaspoons plain gelatin granules
1/2 vanilla bean or 1 teaspoon vanilla extract

Combine the gelatin with 1 tablespoon of warm water in a small bowl. Allow to stand for 10 minutes. In a medium saucepan, heat the cream and maple syrup to medium, whisking continuously to prevent curdling. Allow the mixture to steam slightly, then remove from the heat and allow to cool for five minutes. Whisk in the gelatin mixture until all granules have dissolved completely. Slit the vanilla bean and scrape the contents into the gelatin-cream mixture. Add buttermilk, whisking until the mixture is smooth and creamy. Pour into one large pan or six individual bowls. Refrigerate until firm, 6 hours or more.

*The cream and buttermilk make this recipe unsuitable for paleo dieters.

** Replace the maple syrup with your favorite non-caloric sweeteners to reduce the carbohydrate count of this dessert.

## No-Grain Sandwich Bread (GF, P, LC)

Going grain-free doesn't mean saying goodbye to sandwiches, French toast, bread pudding or stuffing, as long as you know how to use your ingredients. This bread is gluten free and filled with nutrient-dense foods, so you'll be surprised at how satisfying it can be. Fluffy, nutty and light, this bread is everything you dreamed grain-free eating could be!

**Ingredients**

1 3/4 cups almond flour
5 eggs
¼ cup flax seed meal
1/8 cup coconut flour
1 ¾ tablespoons coconut oil
1 tablespoon vinegar
1 tablespoon honey or date paste
1 teaspoon baking soda
¼ teaspoon salt

In a large bowl, combine the almond and coconut flours, flax meal, baking soda and salt. In a separate bowl, whisk together the eggs, coconut oil, vinegar and honey. Pour the wet ingredients into the dry mixture, stirring continuously until just combined. Grease a medium loaf pan and pour the batter in, spreading with a spatula if necessary. Bake at 350 degrees Fahrenheit for 30 minutes or until the top of the loaf browns lightly and the center is firm. Allow to cool and serve.

## Banana Coconut Muffins (GF, P, LC)

These muffins are a delicious treat after dinner or for a quick breakfast on a workday. Their flavor improves a day or so after baking, so don't be afraid to make extra and store them in your refrigerator. The bananas and dates provide plenty of sweetness, so there's no reason to add more carbohydrate-heavy options. If you are in the very-low-carbohydrate phase of a low carb diet, however, these muffins may not be suitable. Try them with a little coconut oil or softened butter, or eat them on their own.

### Ingredients

6 large eggs
3 large bananas
¾ cup coconut flour
½ cup walnuts
5 tablespoons coconut milk
¼ cup coconut oil
2 tablespoons dates
1 tablespoon hot water
2 ½ teaspoons baking powder
½ teaspoon lemon juice
1 teaspoon salt

Soak the dates in the hot water for 10 minutes, then mash with a fork. Combine in a large bowl with the eggs, coconut milk, lemon juice and salt. Stir in coconut oil and set aside. Sift the baking soda and coconut flour into a medium bowl, then stir the dry ingredients slowly into the liquid ones. Mix until no lumps are visible and the ingredients are well mixed.

Peel and mash the bananas, then fold them into the muffin mixture until completely combined. Stir in walnuts. Scoop into a greased 12-cup muffin pan and bake at 400 degrees Fahrenheit for 18 to 20 minutes. Remove from oven and allow to cool for 10 minutes, then release from pan with the tip of a butter knife and enjoy.

## No-flour Chocolate Lava Cake (GF, P)

If you're looking for the perfect holiday dessert indulgence without a trace of grains, this chocolate lava cake is the perfect choice. It includes dark chocolate, which is known for its healthy antioxidants, as well as natural sweeteners. To make ahead, follow the recipe recommendations up to the baking step, then freeze the entire tin and bring to room temperature about a half hour before you bake the cake.

**Ingredients**

½ pound unsweetened baking chocolate
2/3 cup unsalted butter or coconut oil
2/3 cup honey
6 egg yolks
3 egg whites

Combine the chocolate and butter or coconut oil in a heavy-bottomed pot over low heat. In a separate bowl, beat the honey and egg yolks until they are creamy, thick and fluffy. Add the chocolate mixture directly to the egg yolk mixture and beat vigorously for 5 to 10 minutes or until well combined. In a separate container, beat the egg whites until they become frothy and develop stiff peaks. Fold the meringue into the chocolate mixture carefully until just combined. Grease 6 individual ramekins and divide the batter between them. Bake in a 425 degree Fahrenheit oven for 5 to 7 minutes, or until the center is hot and liquid but the edges are solid. Serve hot with your favorite ice cream or frozen yogurt.

## Coconut-vanilla Frozen Dessert (GF, P, LC)

If you read the ingredients on your favorite ice cream package, you may be surprised by how many grain products and fillers it includes. Homemade recipes are often grain-free, but they still rely on refined sugars and other ingredients that tend to be unhealthy. This recipe produces a great-tasting frozen dessert you can make at home without an ice cream maker, plus it's low in carbohydrates and paleo diet-friendly!

**Ingredients**

2 cups coconut milk
2 large eggs
2 vanilla beans or 4 tablespoons vanilla extract
3 tablespoons raw honey or equivalent no-calorie sweetener

Slit the vanilla beans and scrape them thoroughly. Combine the vanilla scrapings with the coconut milk in a double boiler and heat over low heat until steaming. Add the honey or no-calorie sweetener and stir until dissolved. In a separate bowl, whisk the eggs until they are fluffy and thick. Ladle 1/3 to ½ cup of the hot coconut milk mixture into the eggs, whisking vigorously to combine. Repeat the process, then add the egg mixture to the remainder of the coconut milk mixture.

Whisk for 2 to 3 minutes, or until a thick, smooth custard has formed. Remove from heat and allow the custard to cool to room temperature, then transfer to the refrigerator for at least an hour. Pour the custard into a large baking dish and place in the freezer for about 2 hours or until completely set. Stir vigorously to break up the ice once every 15 to 30 minutes. Remove this dessert from the freezer 10 minutes before serving.

## Almond Flour Blueberry Muffins (GF, P, LC*)

This classic snack and breakfast favorite is remarkably simple. It substitutes almond flour for the standard white flour, and natural honey for refined sugar. You'll enjoy the traditional taste, smell and texture of these delicious muffins, whether you eat them fresh out of the oven or save a few for snacking. If your diet doesn't permit use of dairy, consider substituting a grain free soy or coconut yogurt instead.

**Ingredients**

2 ½ cups almond flour
1 cup fresh blueberries
4 tablespoons butter or coconut milk
2 eggs
1/3 cup honey
1/3 cup yogurt
½ vanilla bean or 1 teaspoon vanilla extract
¼ teaspoon nutmeg
¼ teaspoon cinnamon
¼ teaspoon salt

Combine all ingredients other than the blueberries in a large bowl or food processor and beat until well combined. Fold in the blueberries carefully. Grease a 12 cup muffin tin and divide the mixture between the cups. Bake in a 325 degree Fahrenheit oven for 15 to 20 minutes or until the centers have set.

*To make this recipe lower in carbohydrates, substitute your favorite no-calorie sweetener and an equivalent amount of liquid to replace the honey.

## Cinnamon Roll Muffins (GF, P)

Regular cinnamon rolls rely on the gluten found in wheat flour to produce their springy texture and flaky interiors. This muffin recipe duplicates the flavors of cinnamon rolls in muffin form, but it uses no grains. You'll love the rich but healthy taste of their cinnamon topping and the moist interior of these delightful treats.

### Ingredients

1 cup almond flour
¼ cup grapeseed oil
¼ cup agave nectar or maple syrup
1/8 cup coconut flour
3 eggs
1 tablespoon vanilla extract
½ teaspoon baking soda
¼ teaspoon salt
Topping
1/8 cup agave nectar or maple syrup
1 tablespoon coconut oil
1 tablespoon cinnamon

In a medium bowl, combine the flours, salt and baking soda. In a separate large bowl, blend the agave nectar or maple syrup, oil, vanilla extract and eggs. Slowly pour the dry ingredients into the wet mixture, stirring carefully until there are no lumps. Grease a 12 cup muffin tin and spoon batter into the cups. In a small bowl, blend the agave, coconut oil and cinnamon. Divide this mixture between the muffin cups and bake at 350 degrees Fahrenheit for 8 to 12 minutes or until the centers are solid.

## Almond Biscuits (GF, P, LC)

These biscuits have a crisp but crumbly texture and provide plenty of protein. They're great as a part of any breakfast, but they also make an excellent addition to Thanksgiving menus, brunches, dinners and much more. To decrease the carbohydrates in this recipe, simply omit the honey.

### Ingredients

2 ½ cups almond flour
2 eggs
¼ cup coconut oil
1 tablespoon honey
½ teaspoon baking soda
½ teaspoon salt

In a medium bowl, combine the almond flour, soda and salt. In a separate large bowl, blend the eggs, honey and coconut oil. Pour the dry ingredient mixture into the oil mixture, stirring continuously to produce a moldable dough. Place the dough on a piece of parchment paper and cover with an additional piece, then roll out to about 1 ½ inches in thickness. If necessary, dust the dough with additional almond flour.

Using a biscuit cutter or large mouthed glass, cut the

dough into 10 biscuits, rerolling as necessary. Line a baking sheet with parchment paper. Transfer the uncooked biscuits to the sheet using a spatula and bake at 350 degrees Fahrenheit for 15 minutes, or until the bottoms of the biscuits begin to brown. Serve hot with gravy, jam or any other food.

## Rye-style Flax Bread (GF, P, LC)

While a basic sandwich bread works for most uses, not every meal is appropriate for it. That's where a stronger-tasting option can help. This flax seed-based bread has the same color and general flavor as traditional rye bread, but it lacks the potentially-damaging health problems that come with that great. Eat this bread plain, toasted, or as part of your favorite sandwich. To reduce the bread's carbohydrate content, simply omit the honey or replace it with your favorite no-calorie sweetener.

### Ingredients

1 cup almond flour
¾ cup ground flax seed
3 eggs
¼ cup water
2 tablespoons extra virgin olive oil
2 tablespoons caraway seeds
1 teaspoon honey
¾ teaspoon lemon juice
½ teaspoon baking soda
½ teaspoon salt
Coconut oil
Combine the ground flax seed, soda, salt and almond

flour in a large bowl. In a separate small bowl, mix the honey, water, eggs, oil and lemon juice. Slowly stir the wet ingredients into the dry mixture to form a thick batter, then add caraway seeds and mix until evenly distributed. Allow the batter to rest for 5 minutes. Grease a mini loaf pan with coconut oil and fill with the batter. Bake for 30 minutes at 350 degrees Fahrenheit, or until the center is solid. Allow the bread to cool, slice and serve.

# Snacks

## Homemade Yogurt (GF, P, LC*)

Whether you prefer traditional dairy yogurt or you're going milk-free, yogurt is an important staple that any grain-free cook can't do without. It's essential in many baking recipes and makes a delicious meat marinade, as well as a snack on its own. Many commercial yogurts contain large amounts of fillers, sugars and other grain-derived ingredients, making them inappropriate for all kinds of diets. Making your own allows you to control what's in your yogurt and lets you produce the perfect texture for your preferences.

**Ingredients**

4 cups milk, cream or coconut milk
1 tablespoon honey
1 package powdered yogurt starter

Bring the milk, coconut or cream to a boil in a large pot over high heat. Immediately remove from stove and cool to room temperature. Remove 1/2 cup of the liquid to a small separate bowl and combine with the packaged starter. Mix well, then return the starter mixture to the main bowl. Combine thoroughly and pour into a yogurt maker. Ferment for 24 to 30 hours, then remove to the refrigerator to thicken. If desired, strain the yogurt through cheesecloth suspended over a bowl to produce thicker, “Greek-style” yogurt.

*To reduce carbohydrates, omit the honey from dairy-based yogurt. This recipe relies on some sugar for successful fermentation, so no-calorie sweetener is not appropriate.

## Roasted Pumpkin Seeds (GF, P, LC)

These pumpkin seeds with sweet spices are the perfect snack for the autumn holidays. Save the seeds from your jack-o-lantern or pie pumpkins to produce this simple but fragrant food. They're a great substitute for grain-based crackers and unhealthy chips.

### Ingredients

½ cup fresh pumpkin seeds
1 tablespoon olive oil
½ teaspoon ginger powder
¼ teaspoon salt
¼ teaspoon allspice
¼ teaspoon cinnamon
1/8 teaspoon cardamom
1/8 teaspoon cloves
1/8 teaspoon black pepper

In a medium bowl, toss the oil with the pumpkin seeds. In a separate small bowl, combine the powdered spices and stir well. Pour over the seed mixture and stir thoroughly to coat. Bake on an ungreased cookie sheet at 375 degrees Fahrenheit or until fragrant and well-toasted. Eat while still warm or allow to cool. Store in an air-tight container.

## Coconut Chicken Strips (GF, P, LC)

Coconut and chicken are a great combination, and this recipe gives you an alternative to grain-heavy fried snacking options. This baked, non-battered chicken recipe is delicious and a lot of fun to eat, whether it's as a snack or part of a special dinner. Try it with salad, guacamole, or a basic coleslaw recipe.

### Ingredients

1 pound boneless, skinless chicken breasts
1 cup plain shredded coconut
½ cup coconut flour
2 eggs
1 tablespoon coconut milk
1 teaspoon garlic powder
½ teaspoon sharp paprika
salt and black pepper to taste

Flatten the chicken breasts with a mallet or rolling pin to an even thickness. Cut the meat into long pieces approximately 1 inch wide. Combine the eggs, coconut milk, salt and pepper in one small bowl. Beat vigorously until completely mixed. In a separate small bowl, mix the coconut flour, garlic powder and paprika. Place the coconut shreds in a third small bowl.

Working quickly, coat each strip first in coconut flour, then in the egg mixture. Roll the coated strips in shredded coconut and place on a large, ungreased baking sheet. Leave approximately 1 inch between strips. Bake for about 10 minutes at 400 degrees Fahrenheit, or until the chicken is cooked through completely. Eat plain or serve with homemade grain-free plum or sweet and sour sauce.

## Fruit and Nut-Stuffed Pears (GF, P, LC)

Baked pears with sweet spices, rich nuts and fresh fruit is an excellent way to give yourself an energy boost without turning to crackers or cookies. This recipe is natural, healthy, and appropriate for most diets. Very low-carb dieters may find the sugars in the fruit to be excessive, but most should be able to eliminate the honey and still enjoy this treat.

### Ingredients

4 fat, flat-bottomed pears
¼ pound red grapes
¼ cup natural apple juice
2 tablespoons honey
½ cup sliced almonds
½ lemon
1 teaspoon cinnamon

In a small bowl, combine 1 tablespoon of honey with the sliced almonds. Line a baking sheet or pie plate with parchment paper. Bake the almonds on top of the parchment at 300 degrees Fahrenheit for 15 or 20 minutes, or until crisp. Core the pears from the top, leaving the bottom solid. Place the pears on a separate pie plate, cored ends up. Dice the grapes and place them in a small bow. Combine the almond mixture with the grapes and stuff the pears. Juice the lemon and combine it with the apple juice, remaining honey and cinnamon in a small bowl. Pour this mixture into the stuffed cores and all around each piece of fruit. Bake at 300 degrees Fahrenheit for 30 minutes, or until the pears are tender and fully-cooked.

## Sesame Almond Crackers (GF, P, LC)

Chips and crackers make for appealing snacking, but their high percentage of grains and other unhealthy carbohydrates can be damaging to your body. That's why these buttery or coconut-flavored seed-based crackers are such a good alternative. You'll get that savory, crunchy experience you've been craving without the grain.

### Ingredients

¾ cup almond flour
2 tablespoons butter or coconut oil
1 egg white
1 tablespoon sesame seeds
3/8 teaspoon salt
¼ teaspoon onion powder
¼ teaspoon garlic powder

Beat the egg white until frothy. Allow the butter to soften at room temperature. In a small bowl, combine all dry ingredients, then blend in egg white and butter until a soft dough forms. Chill for 30 minutes, then drop by ¼ teaspoons onto a baking sheet lined with parchment. Leave 1 inch or more between dough balls. Cover with parchment paper or plastic wrap and flatten to about 1/16 inch thick. Prick with a fork and bake for 20 minutes at 325 degrees Fahrenheit, or until golden brown. Allow to cool and store in an airtight container.

## Cheese Crisps (GF, P*, LC)

Crispy, crunchy and composed entirely of cheese, these unique little snacks are a grain-free dieter's snacking salvation. They're low in carbohydrates and high in flavor, making them a satisfying choice for between-meal treats. Try several different kinds of cheese to make a variety mix. Plus, these simple crisps can be made in the microwave!

**Ingredients**

8 ounce bag shredded cheddar, mozzarella, Swiss or Monterey jack cheese
garlic powder or onion powder to taste (optional)

Line a microwaveable plate or tray with parchment paper. Place 1 tablespoon of shredded cheese in the middle of the plate and spread it out into an even layer approximately 3 inches across. Microwave on high for 30 seconds. Remove the paper and crisp from the plate and allow it to cool, then peel the paper off of the crisp. Repeat using the same piece of parchment paper. When all crisps are cool, store in an air-tight container. For longer storage, try the freezer.

*Paleo dieters may need to eat these in moderation, as

some diets restrict dairy.

## Chicken Cracklings (GF, P, LC)

These meaty snacks may sound a little unusual at first, but they'll soon grow on you. They're made using the same theory as pork rinds, but without the pig. The result is salty, meaty and surprisingly low in “bad” fats. This recipe is also great for using the skin from chicken thigh recipes that require skinless meat.

**Ingredients**

Skin from 8 pre-roasted chicken thighs
Salt and pepper to taste

Cut the pieces of skin into pieces a few inches across and spread them in a single layer on a large baking sheet. Avoid stacking the skins, as this can prevent crisping. Season lightly with salt on one side and bake for 30 minutes at 350 degrees Fahrenheit. Flip the skin and bake an additional 10 minutes, or until crisp and brown. Eat immediately or allow the cracklings to cool and store in the refrigerator. Reheat before serving.

# Salads, Soups and Sides

## Creamy Cauliflower Soup (GF, P, LC)

This rich and delicious soup makes a great substitute for potato or grain-based soups on a chilly day. It's also egg free, for diets that limit egg consumption. Substitute vegetable stock for the chicken stock to make this dish vegetarian-friendly for larger gatherings or guests.

1 head cauliflower
2 quarts chicken stock
1 large onion
¼ cup milk
2 tablespoons olive oil
1 teaspoons them
salt and pepper to taste

Chop the onion and the cauliflower. Mince the garlic. Heat the olive oil in a large pot over medium heat and sauté the onion and garlic for 5 minutes, or until translucent. Add the stock, thyme and cauliflower, then bring to a boil over high heat. Reduce to a simmer and cook until the cauliflower almost dissolves. Puree in a blender until completely smooth, then season with salt and pepper as desired. Serve hot, garnished with thyme.

## Matzoh Ball Soup (GF, P, LC)

This traditional Passover soup is also beloved by plenty of non-Jewish cooks. It's known as a health-boosting remedy for cold or flu, but the wheat-based matzoh it requires is off-limits for grain-free diets. This version uses almond flour instead of wheat flour to produce surprisingly authentic-tasting matzoh balls. Whether you'd like a wheat-free substitute for your Passover table or you just love chicken soup, this recipe will soon be staple of your cookbook. To render the soup vegetarian-friendly, simply substitute vegetable broth instead of chicken.

**Ingredients**

6 cups chicken stock
2 cups almond flour
4 eggs
2 teaspoons salt
pepper to taste

Combine eggs, salt and pepper in a medium bowl, beating vigorously. Slowly add the almond flour, stirring continuously to produce a soft dough. Refrigerate for at least 2 hours and set aside. Boil a large pot of water over high heat and drop the batter by tablespoons-full into the boiling liquid. Reduce heat to low, cover, and allow to simmer for 20 minutes. Remove with a slotted spoon. In a separate pot, heat 6 cups chicken stock to a simmer. Gently place the finished matzoh balls into the stock and heat for an additional 10 minutes. Serve hot, with at least 2 to 3 matzoh balls per bowl.

## Split Pea and Mushroom Soup (GF)

This hearty soup provides protein in the form of mushrooms and split peas, savory flavors from stock, garlic and onion, and a little spice in the form of paprika. This recipe contains no meat, but if you'd like more of a meaty flavor, substitute chicken or beef stock for the vegetable broth. Like many hearty soups, this recipe is actually best the next day.

### Ingredients

1 quart vegetable broth
3 cups water
1 cup split yellow peas
½ pound mushrooms
1 cup kale
2 tablespoons olive oil
2 cloves garlic
1 small onion
2 bay leaves
½ teaspoon smoked paprika
salt and black pepper to taste

Combine bay leaves, split peas, water and paprika in a medium pan. Bring to a boil over high heat, then reduce to low and simmer until the peas fall apart. Remove from heat and set aside. Discard bay leaves. Chop onions, kale and garlic. In a large pan, heat the olive oil to medium-low and sauté chopped onion. Slice the mushrooms and add to the pan with the garlic and kale. Cook until tender and set aside. Remove bay leaf from split peas. Combine pea mixture with mushroom mixture along with stock. Cook for 30 minutes or until thick and well combined. Serve hot.

## Squash Oven Fries (GF, P, LC)

Even for potato eaters, conventional fries tend to be off-limits for a grain-free diet because of the risk that they have been cooked in corn oil. These lower-carbohydrate substitutes are made from squash, cooked in olive oil, and made right in your home oven. They're crisp and much healthier. Choose them as a side for your next batch of barbecue chicken or even to go with your morning eggs.

### Ingredients

1 large butternut squash or pumpkin
¼ cup olive oil
1 tablespoon dried oregano
salt and black pepper to taste

Cut the squash in half lengthwise and remove the seeds. Peel the outside and cut the meat into sticks of your preferred size. Place the squash fries in a large bowl and toss them with the olive oil, then the spices. Season to taste with salt and pepper. Place in a single layer on a large cookie sheet and roast at 425 degrees Fahrenheit for 20 minutes, or until the outside is crisp.

## Cranberry Steak Salad (GF, P, LC)

This salad is hearty enough to be a meal in and of itself. It uses skirt steak, which is not normally considered a tender or appealing cut, but careful preparation helps bring out the incredible flavors of this meat. When combined with fresh cranberries and fennel, it produces a fresh salad that's affordable and delicious. If fresh cranberries are unavailable in your area, consider substituting frozen.

1 pound skirt steak
2 cups arugula
1 large bulb fennel
½ cup fresh cranberries
2 scallions
1 tablespoon olive oil
1 tablespoon fresh thyme
1 tablespoon fresh basil
1 bunch flat leaf parsley
salt and pepper to taste
3 tablespoons of your favorite vinaigrette

Fill a small pot with water and bring it to a boil over high heat. Add the cranberries and cook for about 5 minutes, or until the berries soften. Drain and set aside to cool. Season the steak with salt and black pepper to taste, then sprinkle thoroughly with basil and thyme. Heat the coconut oil in a large skillet over medium-high heat and add the steak. Cook, flipping frequently throughout the process, until the steak reaches your preferred level of doneness. Transfer to a plate or cutting board and allow to rest for 5 minutes.

Slice the fennel thinly and combine in a large bowl with the cranberries and arugula. Cut the steak into thin slices and toss with the vegetables. Serve topped with your favorite dressing and garnish with parsley.

## Spinach and Blood Orange Salad (GF, P)

Light and refreshing, this salad is a delicious starter or small meal. The fruit adds tartness and sweetness, while the spinach provides plenty of important minerals. Combined with honey and almonds, this recipe is a great meatless addition to just about any meal. If you can't obtain blood oranges, consider substituting Meyer lemons or sweet pink grapefruit.

### Ingredients

½ cup spinach leaves
2 medium blood oranges
1 sweet pear
½ cup slivered or chopped almonds
¼ cup dried, unsweetened cranberries
1 tablespoon honey
Dressing
½ cup olive oil
2 tablespoons rice vinegar
1 teaspoon prepared brown mustard
salt and pepper to taste

In a small bowl, combine the honey with the almonds. Line a baking sheet with parchment paper and spread the almonds over it. Bake at 300 degrees Fahrenheit for

15 to 20 minutes or until browned. Remove and set aside.

In a separate bowl, combine the olive oil, rice vinegar, mustard, salt and pepper. Whisk vigorously to combine and set aside. Cut the pear and citrus fruit into large pieces. Combine in a large bowl with the spinach and dried cranberries. Pour the vinaigrette over the entire salad and toss. Serve garnished with honeyed almonds.

## Kale Coleslaw (GF, P, LC)

Traditional cabbage coleslaw is perfectly appropriate for a grain-free diet, as long as you can ensure that the dressing includes no dextrose or other grain-derived ingredients. This recipe provides a little extra punch, however. It includes nutrient-dense kale and almonds, making it much healthier than the standard fare.

### Ingredients

2 large bunches kale
1 pound carrots
2 scallions
½ cup olive oil
½ cup coconut oil
¼ cup chopped almonds
2 egg yolks
1 tablespoon lemon juice
1 tablespoon prepared mustard
salt and pepper to taste

Cut the kale and scallions into thin strips. Shred the carrots and toss with the kale mixture. Mix in the almonds, stirring carefully. Mix the olive and coconut oils together in a small pan or microwaveable bowl and heat until just melted. In a small bowl, combine the egg yolks, mustard and 1 teaspoon of the lemon juice. Whisk vigorously, dripping the melted oils in slowly to create an emulsion. Stabilize the bowl with a cloth or towel if necessary. When the dressing reaches the desired consistency, add the remaining lemon juice. Season with salt and pepper. Add 2 or 3 tablespoons of dressing to the kale mixture and stir to coat. Refrigerate and serve cold.

## Roasted Winter Squash (GF, P, LC)

This simple side dish is tasty and appropriate for a wide range of diet restrictions. It's gluten-free, contains no dairy, and also lacks meat. Some low-carbohydrate diets prohibit winter squash, but this mildly-sweet dish should be appropriate for the later stages of these eating plans. Enjoy roasted squash as a side with your favorite meats or on its own as a light meal.

### Ingredients

1 acorn squash or 2 delicata squash
¼ cup olive or coconut oil
1 teaspoon cinnamon
salt and pepper to taste

Cut the squash in half lengthwise and remove the stems, seeds and membranes. Place cut side down on a cutting board and cut into slices about ¼ inch thick. Lay in a single layer on a large cookie sheet, leaving space between each piece. Drizzle with 1/8 cup oil, then sprinkle with salt, pepper and cinnamon. Bake at 400 degrees Fahrenheit for 10 minutes, or until golden brown. Flip, drizzle with the remaining oil, and bake for an additional 5 minutes. Serve hot.

# A 5-Day Grain Free Meal Plan

This sample grain free meal plan is designed to help you get an idea of the best way to go grain free. It is not oriented toward any one type of diet, however. That means that if you need to avoid specific ingredients, it may be necessary to modify the meal plan slightly. Use this diet plan as a springboard for your new way of cooking, rather than an exact set of rules. After all, there's nothing to limit you other than your imagination!

**Day 1**

Breakfast: Hot Porridge, orange juice

Lunch: Cranberry Steak Salad

Snack: Cheese Crisps, sliced pears

Dinner: Braised Chicken with Sweet Potatoes and Fennel Bulb, Spinach and Blood Orange Salad

**Day 2**

Breakfast: Green Eggs, Rye-style Flax Bread

Lunch: Split Pea and Mushroom Soup

Snack: Homemade Yogurt

Dinner: Stuffed Bell Peppers with Veal, Kale Coleslaw

**Day 3**

Breakfast: Banana Coconut Muffins

Lunch: American Taco Pie

Snack: Cinnamon Roll Muffins

Dinner: Pot Roast with Fresh Vegetables, Almond Biscuits

**Day 4**

Breakfast: Sweet Potato Breakfast Casserole

Lunch: Roasted Winter Squash, Coconut Chicken Strips

Snack: Fruit and Nut-Stuffed Pears

Dinner: Creamy Cauliflower Soup, Barbecue Chicken with Grain-free Sauce

**Day 5**

Breakfast: Almond Waffles, orange juice, Homemade Yogurt

Lunch: Baked Cashew Chicken

Snack: Roasted Pumpkin Seeds

Dinner: Zucchini Pasta with Roasted Sweet Potatoes and Coconut Pesto, Squash Oven Fries, Coconut-vanilla Frozen Dessert

# Conclusion

There's no reason to feel like eating grain-free has to be a limitation. The world is full of fantastic and healthy grain-free recipes that are suitable for paleo dieters, celiacs and other with wheat sensitivities, and low-carb eating plans. If you just take a little bit of time to think about all the options, you'll be surprised by all the great things you can eat. While it can be difficult living in a wheat and corn-obsessed world, you won't be in danger of going hungry. All you have to do with learn to think outside the grain-based box.

These recipes provide a starting place for anyone who wants to enjoy their food without worrying about the health problems that grains and other carbohydrates could be causing. It's time to stop suffering from headaches, digestive problems, nutritional deficiencies and all the other issues that modern grains can induce. The alternatives are rich, delicious and extremely healthy. Try a new no-grain recipe today!